II 010672
1600

C0-BLD-345

CRITICAL CARE MANUAL

A SYSTEMS APPROACH METHOD

SECOND EDITION

By

BURTON A. WAISBREN, M.D., F.A.C.P.
Internist and Associate Director
of St. Mary's Hospital Burn Center

Director, St. Mary's Hospital Burn Research
and Clinical Paradigm Laboratory

Founding Member, American Burn Association

Associate Clinical Professor of Medicine,
Medical College of Wisconsin

Member of the Board and Founding Member,
American Society of Critical Care Medicine

Member of Critical Care Committee,
St. Mary's Hospital,
Milwaukee, Wisconsin

Member of Emergency Care Council,
American Heart Association

Founding Member, Infectious Disease Society of America

Director, The Clinical Cell Biology Laboratory of
Mount Sinai Medical Center

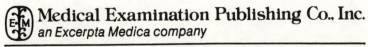
Medical Examination Publishing Co., Inc.
an Excerpta Medica company

969 Stewart Avenue • Garden City, New York 11530

notice ━━━━━━━━

The editor(s) and/or author(s) and the publisher of this book have made every effort
to ensure that all therapeutic modalities
that are recommended are in accordance
with accepted standards at the time of publication.

The drugs specified within this book may
not have specific approval by the Food and
Drug Administration in regard to the indications and dosages that are recommended
by the editor(s) and/or author(s).   The
manufacturer's package insert is the best
source of current prescribing information.

Copyright © 1977 by
MEDICAL EXAMINATION
PUBLISHING CO., INC.

Library of Congress Card Number
77-71847

ISBN 0-87488-983-9

May, 1977

All rights reserved. No part of this
publication may be reproduced in any
form or by any means, electronic or
mechanical, including photocopy,
without permission in writing from
the publisher.

Printed in the United States of America

PREFACE TO THE SECOND EDITION

It is gratifying indeed to be able to write a second edition of this Manual. In this new edition I have tried to match the spotty progress of most institutions toward computerization by presenting the information in such a way that it can go directly into the total information systems of the most advanced hospitals but still be completely understandable to those hospitals that are still using trusty humans as their computers (See chapter on computerization, page 222).

Because I use most of the methods outlined in this Manual almost every day, I have been surprised at how revolutionary they seem to some of my fellow clinicians. Accordingly, I have included several chapters in which the conceptual basis of our approach is discussed (Chapter - Essays - pages 222-255).

Suggestions that I have received have been incorporated into the manual, and I again ask for suggestions for future editions.

I have kept the single author format and remain responsible for all opinions expressed. However, my debt to my colleagues, both in the nursing and medical professions at the St. Mary's Burn Center and in the Critical Care Units in the Milwaukee area, is apparent and I wish to thank them all for their help, support, and criticisms.

Special thanks and appreciation have been earned by my secretary and associate, Mrs. Enid Reichert, who did far more than typing in getting this Manual together.

PREFACE TO FIRST EDITION

CONCEPTUAL BASIS FOR THE CRITICAL CARE
FLOWSHEET CONTINGENCY ORDER MANUAL

Many clinical decisions are made almost automatically upon receipt of crucial laboratory values. In this Manual we have tried to analyze this process and present it in a manner that would allow trained paramedical personnel to administer needed medications and procedures without the delay that often ensues if the physician in charge has to be located before an affirmative action is taken.

Even though there is a growing tendency to group the most seriously ill patients in a hospital in an Intensive Care area, it is unlikely in the near future that the majority of critically ill patients in the United States will have a trained physician in constant attendance. Furthermore, physicians are in too short supply for them to be sitting around Critical Care Units waiting for something to happen. They can better spend their time in the Library or in providing primary care.

Thus, it is hoped that Manuals of this type will allow better treatment of this majority of critically ill patients by affording a means by which the proper reactions to change in their condition can be more promptly and efficiently noted without the necessity of constant M.D. attendance.

The critically ill patients, during whose treatment this Manual was developed, were suffering from severe burns, gram-negative shock, overwhelming pneumonia, cardiogenic shock, postoperative complications, and severe trauma. Many controversial methods and actions are presented in this Manual, and time and the reader's own experiences will decide their ultimate validity. However, each value decision made by the author in the Manual was based on his personal experience in treating, on the average, a critically ill patient each day for the past twenty-five years.

CRITICAL CARE MANUAL
Second Edition

CONTENTS

THIS MANUAL IS DEDICATED

TO

FLORENCE

DISCLAIMER

All suggestions in this Manual are the personal, considered opinions of the author. Responsibility for what happens to any individual patient who is treated on the basis of this Manual remains with the physician who activates the order. In addition, the reader should check with his own laboratory normals and make appropriate corrections in the Manual.

DEFINITIONS, CHALLENGE, AND AN INVITATION TO ADOPT FORMS

CRITICAL ILLNESS is defined in this Manual as a potentially reversible illness that has a good chance of killing the patient within 48 hours.

CRITICAL CARE is defined as the total management of a patient while he is suffering a critical illness.

CHALLENGE: Each Intensive Care Unit ought to be able to improve each page of this Manual and we challenge you to do this.

ALL ideas for improvement that are sent to the author and incorporated in the next edition will be suitably acknowledged.

FEEL FREE TO COPY AND USE as many forms and flowsheets in the Manual as you think may be of help to you in caring for your patients, just as I have felt free to share with you many forms and flowsheets that have come to my attention.

USE OF THE MANUAL AS A PROCEDURE GUIDE FOR
A CRITICAL CARE OR INTENSIVE CARE UNIT

The Accreditation bodies at this point tend to judge Critical Care Units on the basis of their written procedure guides. This Manual can be utilized as it is for a Procedure Guide, providing that the physicians and nurses responsible for the patients in the Unit go over it and agree on the way this should be done. Material written on blank pages will provide for adaption to local problems and for opinions differing from those of the author.

USE OF THE MANUAL FOR TEACHING

With this Manual on the desk a nurse or physician should be able to take any patient's chart and figure out the whys and wherefores of the treatment. He can first go through all the laboratory work and look up the meaning of all abnormal values; and then go through the FAIL-SAFE drug section and see why each medication is being given and how the patient is being protected from possible toxic effects of the drugs he is receiving.

ALTERNATIVE SUGGESTIONS TO THE NURSES AND ADMINISTRATION FOR IMPLEMENTATION OF THE CRITICAL CARE SYSTEM TECHNIQUES AS PRESENTED IN THIS MANUAL

1. TRAIN non-nursing personnel to retrieve data from the laboratory as soon as it is obtainable and to place these values on the flowsheet, with instructions to bring to the CRITICAL CARE nurse's attention any values outside the normal range. These personnel can write requisitions for CONTINGENCY ORDER laboratory work, i.e., for studies to be done on the patient on the basis of returned laboratory work. Used in this manner, the Manual can be used in the absence of any of the computer techniques we discuss so often--by using the best computer for them all--a human brain attached to an interested ward secretary, or as we call them, a Ward Communicator.

OR

2. HAVE a prior agreement with the attending physicians as to which CONTINGENCY ORDERS, of both diagnostic and therapeutic type, should be automatically operative.

OR

3. DO a prospective study of "what we would have done" with the Manual as compared with "what we did" with your present system to decide whether or not this Manual has potential help for your patients and then decide whether all concerned feel that a System in the Intensive Care Unit should have been adopted.

OR

4. HAVE a System--as outlined in the Manual and as modified by the Intensive Care Committee--accepted through the whole committee structure of the hospital staff. Then make the entire modified manual specifically operative.

AND

5. DO NOT DO ANYTHING SUGGESTED IN THIS MANUAL IF--AT THE TIME--IT VIOLATES YOUR COMMON SENSE.

HOW TO IMPLEMENT THE SYSTEMS AND THE ORDERS

The Standing Order Sheets which follow can either be ordered by the physician over the phone, or initialled in person, or first ordered by phone and then initialled.

Before the reader considers the laboratory monitoring excessive, he should remember our definition regarding who should be a patient in a Critical Care Unit-- one who is in <u>imminent danger of death.</u>

The Order Sheet is the means by which the patient's personal physician remains in <u>direct control</u> of the patient, since order numbers 25, 26, 27 and 28 (page 16) give him three options:

1. Use of <u>ALL</u> Contingency Orders accepted by his Critical Care Committee or Department. (He checks 27.)

OR

2. Use of <u>only</u> DIAGNOSTIC Contingency Orders. (He checks 26.)

OR

3. The option of having <u>only</u> direct new orders honored. (He checks 28.)

In addition to the 8-hour-shift Critical Care Flowsheet (page 25) the patient's physician can have any other specialty flowsheet kept up that he feels will make it easier for him to manage his patient. (pages 21, 23, 25, 27, 29, 41, 43, 45, 47, and 49)

SUGGESTED ORDER SHEET

The nurse can get instructions by reading this to the physician by phone or he can check or initial it on the spot.

CHECK OR INITIAL: **ORDERS:**

☐ 1. Light on at all times.

☐ 2. Family may be at bedside.

☐ 3. May be taken to safe area to smoke.

☐ 4. May have telephone.

☐ 5. May have usual dose of following laxatives upon preference and request and may use several if one does not work: milk of magnesia, mineral oil, Dulcolax, or Dulcolax suppository.

☐ 6. Diet -- regular.

☐ 7. Diet -- low salt.

☐ 8. Diet -- N.P.O.

☐ 9. Diet -- select.

☐ 10. Diet -- other.

☐ 11. Have priest see patient for last rites.

☐ 12. Sedation -- chloral hydrate, $7\frac{1}{2}$ gr., H.S. p.r.n., if <u>over</u> age 60.

☐ 13. Sedation -- seconal, gr. 1ss., H.S.. p.r.n., if <u>under</u> age 60.

☐ 14. Pain relief -- none.

☐ 15. Pain relief -- demerol, ____ mg. every 6 hours.

☐ 16. Pain relief -- morphine, ____ every 6 hours.

☐ 17. Pain relief -- other _____.

☐ 18. CRITICAL CARE PACKAGE: CBC, reticulocyte count, blood gases, Na, K, Ca, platelet count, chest x-ray, serum and urine osmolalities, and 12-hour creatinine clearance. If fever is present or wound is draining, culture blood, sputum, drainage, and urine. Get digoxin level if patient is receiving digoxin or cedilanid.

16

FREQUENCY OF CRITICAL CARE PACKAGE:

☐ 19. Daily.

☐ 20. Mondays, Wednesdays, and Fridays.

☐ 21. When ordered.

☐ 22. NO cardiopulmonary resuscitation to be attempted.

☐ 23. Cardiopulmonary resuscitation to point of fixed pupils.

☐ 24. Cardiopulmonary resuscitation for only 10 minutes.

☐ 25. In addition to CRITICAL CARE PACKAGE get blood alcohol, carbon monoxide, barbiturate, and drug levels.

☐ 26. Activate all DIAGNOSTIC CONTINGENCY ORDERS as modified by CRITICAL CARE COMMITTEE of the hospital, based on abnormal values of Critical Care Flowsheet.

☐ 27. Activate all DIAGNOSTIC AND CONTINGENCY ORDERS as modified by CRITICAL CARE COMMITTEE of the hospital, based on abnormal values of Critical Care Flowsheet.

☐ 28. All orders will be given directly.

FLOWSHEETS TO BE KEPT UP

☐ 29. Contingency Order Flowsheet - with cardiac values (page 21).

☐ 30. Contingency Order Flowsheet - without cardiac values (page 23).

☐ 31. Eight-hour shift Critical Care Flowsheet (page 25).

☐ 32. Daily Trend Assisted Ventilation Flowsheet (page 27).

☐ 33. Heart Status and Ventricular Function Flowsheet.

☐ 34. Suspected Coronary Flowsheet (page 41).

☐ 35. Hyperalimentation Flowsheet (page 45).

☐ 36. Dialysis Flowsheet (page 47).

☐ 37. Immunodepressed or Cancer Chemotherapy Flowsheet (page 49).

☐ 38. Bleeding Diathesis Flowsheet (page 43).

SYSTEMS TO BE INSTITUTED

☐   39.   Antibiotic Treatment of Infection System (page 142).

☐   40.   Chest X-ray Findings System (page 151).

☐   41.   Assisted Ventilation System (page 155).

☐   42.   Stress Ulcer System (page 161).

☐   43.   Dialysis System (page 163).

☐   44.   Swan-Ganz System (page 169).

☐   45.   Shock Lung System (page 172).

☐   46.   Hypovolemic System (page 173).

☐   47.   Cardiogenic Shock System (page 179).

☐   48.   Gram-negative Shock System (page 174).

☐   49.   Cardiac Shock System (page 176).

☐   50.   Potassium Control System (page 177).

☐   51.   Anaphylactic Shock System (page 180).

☐   52.   Single Life Line Intravenous Support System (page 181).

☐   53.   Hyperalimentation System (page 184).

☐   54.   Fever of Unknown Etiology System (page 187).

☐   55.   Pulmonary Embolism System (page 189).

☐   56.   Prevention of Fat Embolism System (page 190).

☐   57.   Drug FAIL-SAFE System (page 191).

☐   58.   Digitalis System (page 196).

☐   59.   Intra-aortic Balloon Pumping System (page 199).

☐   60.   Coumadin Anticoagulation System (page 200).

☐   61.   Heparin Anticoagulation System (page 203).

☐   62.   Bleeding Diathesis System (page 204).

☐   63.   Compromised Host System (page 205).

18

64. Diabetic Coma and/or Diabetic Hyperglycemia, Hyperosmolality, and Lactic Acidosis System (page 209).

ADDITIONAL MEDICATIONS -- PARENTERAL:

MONITORING AND MACHINES

DO	STAND BY	
☐	☐	EKG -- Visual Continual Monitor.
☐	☐	CVP every 2 hours.
☐	☐	Pulmonary artery and wedge pressure.
☐	☐	Standby pacing.
☐	☐	Cardiac output.
☐	☐	Hyperbaric oxygen.
☐	☐	Balloon pump.

OPTIONS REGARDING CONTINGENCY ORDERS

The orders and discussion that follow are to be used as directed by the physicians on the ORDER SHEET (page 16, Orders Nos. 25, 26, 27, 28, 29, 31 and 32).

To find the proper CONTINGENCY ORDER look for the correct page number opposite the normal range of the laboratory value that is abnormal on the CONTINGENCY ORDER FLOWSHEET (pages 21 and 23). For instance, if the ApO_2 is < 70 the ward secretary should be turned to for explanations and orders, depending on the method chosen by the physician on page

On the CONTINGENCY ORDER pages we have tried to give simple, helpful explanations of what might be happening to the patient.

ADDITIONAL STANDING ORDERS
AS DETERMINED BY INDIVIDUAL UNITS

CONTINGENCY ORDER FLOWSHEET — WITH CARDIAC MONITORING VALUES

Admission Date		**Hospital Day**						
Weight in Kilos — > 250 see page 51								
Age < 10 or > 65 (page 52)								
Weight Changes ± 3 change (page 52)								
Urine Output > 4000 or < 1000 (page)								

IF VALUES
ON FLOWSHEET
ARE IN
RANGE OF
CONTINGENCY
ORDERS – – –
TURN TO PAGE
INDICATED IN
PAGE COLUMN
FOR ORDERS &
EXPLANATION

INTAKE — LITERS
I.V. & ORAL

OUTPUT — LITERS
I.F.L.* (page 54)
URINE (pages 55-57)
G.I. TRACT

12
10
8
6
4
2

2
4
6
8

CONTINGENCY ORDER LEVEL	SEE PAGES							
Fluid Balance > 4000 or < 4000	Pages 55, 57, 59, 60							
pAO_2 < 70	61							
$pACO_2$ > 45 or < 25	63-65							
HCO_3 < 22 or > 36	66-67							
Lactic acid > 2.8	68							
Base excess ± 3	69							
pH < 7.3 or > 7.5	71							
pAO_2 c̄ 100% O_2 by mask — daily change of 10	73-75							
Shunt percentage increasing	75							
Tidal volume < 500	77							
Blood pressure > 250 or < 90	81, 83, 85							
Blood volume > 75 ml/kilo or < 45 ml/kilo	78, 79							
Pulmonary artery diastolic pressure < 3 or > 18	87, 84							
Pulmonary artery systolic pressure > 28	30, 31, 87, 89							
Wedge pressure > 18 or + 5 change in one hour	91, 92							
Peripheral resistance > 2000	93							
AO_2 Sat-VO_2 Sat — 10 difference	30, 31, 70							
Cardiac index < 4 or > 10	30, 31, 95, 96							
Digoxin level < 1.5 or > 2.5	97							
Hematocrit < 20 hemoglobin < 10.5	101							
WBC > 15000 or < 3500	103-104							
Fibrinogen < 250	109							
Prothrombin time > 15 sec. or < 40%	111, 193, 200							
Platelet count < 80,000	105							
Reticulocyte count < .3	107							
SGPT > 30	98							
Serum bilirubin > 2	99							
BUN < 10 or > 20	113, 115							
Creatinine clearance < 60 or decrease of 20	117							
Serum osmolality > 350 or < 315	119							
Urine osmolality < 250	121							
Na > 150 or < 130	123, 125							
K < 3.8 or > 5.5	127, 129							
Calcium < 7 or > 10	131, 132							
Blood sugar < 80 or > 300	133, 135							
Temperature > 104° or < 96°	138							
Stabs 65% or over 20% rise	139							
Cortisol < 5	137							
Culture { Urine Blood Wound } { E = E. coli, P = Proteus, K = Klebsiella, Ps = Pseudo., S = Staph. }	141 TO 149							
EKG x = change	212-219							
Chest x-ray x = change	151-153							

*I.F.L. = Insensible Fluid Loss

<u>NOTES</u>

CONTINGENCY ORDER FLOWSHEET — WITHOUT CARDIAC MONITORING VALUES

Age (see page 51)		Hospital Day							
Weight in Kilos (see page 52) ±3 lb. change									

| IF VALUES ON FLOWSHEET ARE IN RANGE OF CONTINGENCY ORDERS — — — TURN TO PAGE INDICATED IN PAGE COLUMN FOR ORDERS & EXPLANATION | INTAKE — LITERS I.V. & ORAL | 12 10 8 6 4 2 | | | | | | | |
| | OUTPUT — LITERS I.F.L.* (page 54) URINE (pages 55-60) G.I. TRACT | 2 4 6 8 | | | | | | | |

CONTINGENCY ORDER LEVEL	SEE PAGES							
Fluid Balance > 4000 or < 4000	Pages 55, 57, 59, 60							
pAO_2 < 70	61							
$pACO_2$ > 45 or < 25	63, 65							
HCO_3 < 22 or > 36	66, 67							
Lactic acid > 2.8	68							
Base excess ± 3	69							
pH < 7.3 or > 7.5	71							
pAO_2 c̄ 100% O_2 by mask — daily change of 10	30, 31 73, 75							
Shunt percentage increasing	75							
Tidal volume < 500	77							
Blood pressure > 250 or < 90	81, 83, 85							
Blood volume > 75 ml/kilo or < 45 ml/kilo	78, 79							
Digoxin level < 1.5 or > 2.5	97							
Hematocrit < 20 hemoglobin < 10.5	101							
WBC > 1500 or < 3500	103-104							
Fibrinogen < 250	109							
Prothrombin time > 15 sec. or < 40%	111, 193, 200							
Platelet count < 80,000	105							
Reticulocyte count < .3	107							
SGPT > 30	98							
Serum bilirubin > 2	99							
BUN < 10 or > 20	113, 115							
Creatinine clearance < 60 or decrease of 20	117							
Serum osmolality > 350 or < 315	119							
Urine osmolality < 250	121							
Na > 150 or < 130	123, 125							
K < 3.8 or > 5.5	127, 129							
Calcium < 7 or > 10	131, 132							
Blood sugar < 80 or > 300	133, 135							
Temperature > 104° or < 96°	138							
Stabs 65% or over 20% rise	139							
Cortisol < 5	137							
Culture { Urine Blood Wound } { E = E. coli / P = Proteus / K = Klebsiella / Ps = Pseudo. / S = Staph. }	141 TO 149							
EKG x = change	212-219							
Chest x-ray x = change	151-153							

*I.F.L. = Insensible Fluid Loss

NOTES

8 HR. SHIFT CRITICAL CARE FLOW SHEET

TIME										TIME			

TEMPERATURE X: 104 103 102 101 100 99 98 97

BLOOD PRESSURE symbol-∧ or-∨ — **PULSE** symbol-o: 190 180 170 160 150 140 130 120 110 100 90 80 70 60 50 40 30

PULMONARY ARTERY PRESSURE Systolic∧ Diastolic∨ Wedge o: 28 26 24 22 20 18 16 14 12 10 8 6 4 2

Right labels: Hgb, Hct, Na, K, ApO$_2$, VpO$_2$, Osmol, BUN, Creat, Glucose, CPK, SGOT, LDH, SGPT, CT, Pro T, Na, K

DOCTORS VISITED:

ACTIVITY:

FLUID BALANCE — OUT: SP GR, URINE, STOOL, GI, BLOOD LOSS, OTHER — IN: BLOOD IN, IV, ORAL, OTHER

TOTALS | TOTAL OUT | WEIGHT | TOTAL IN | + | −

SIGNS: EKG, CNS, COLOR, SKIN TEMP, R R, O$_2$

DIET:

APPETITE:

SIGNATURES:

NOTES

ASSISTED VENTILATION FLOWSHEET

Name			
Date			
Hospital day			
	Value		
1.	Rate		
2.	Tidal volume		
3.	Inspiration		
4.	Expiration		
5.	Concentration of O_2		
6.	PEEP/CPAP		
7.			
8.			
9.			
10.			
11.			
12.			
13.			
14.			
15.			

1.	ApO_2 PaO_2	
2.	pCO_2	
3.	pH	
4.	HCO_3	
5.	Base excess	
6.	BUN	
7.	Chest x-ray	
8.	Na	
9.	K	
10.	Cl	
11.		
12.		
13.		
14.		
15.		

CONCEPTUAL BASIS OF REACTIONS TO INFORMATION
ON CARDIAC FUNCTION FLOW SHEETS

Therapy must be concerned with maintaining cardiac output. <u>First</u> consideration here is adequate blood volume. We use Starling's law to do this, <u>i. e.</u>, more tension, more contractible force up to a point. Therefore, at a minimum, there must be a pulmonary artery diastolic pressure of 5. This can be increased by increasing rate of fluid administration as long as this causes an increase in cardiac output.

<u>Second</u>, when maximum cardiac output has been achieved by fluid administration (assuming always that patient is digitalized to level of 2. 5), attention to blood pressure is next. If blood pressure is under 100, this can be increased by an ionotropic agent such as norepinephrine or dopamine. These agents can be counterproductive if they push up blood pressure but also increase peripheral resistance. Therefore, peripheral vasodilators, such as sodium nitroprusside (Nipride), must be used with ionotropic agents to keep peripheral resistance under 2000.

<u>Third</u>, fluids, digitalis, and ionotropic agents should only be used to the point that they do not increase heart work. When heart work starts to go up markedly, they can be counterproductive, especially when there has been a myocardial infarction, which may, in this set of circumstances, increase its area due to the increased work.

CARDIAC FUNCTION MONITORING FLOWSHEET

The advent of thermodilution cardiac output through the Swan-Ganz catheter makes possible meticulous monitoring of cardiac function through the simple expedient of injecting some cold D5W into the pulmonary readout--and then using the nomograms on pages 32, 33, 35, 37 and 39 to fill in the Cardiac Function Flowsheet.

CARDIAC FUNCTION FLOWSHEET

Reading By Either Daily or Hourly Sequences

Determination	Range	Nomogram Page				
Systemic Blood Pressure						
Mean Blood Pressure						
Pulmonary Artery Blood Pressure						
Wedge Blood Pressure						
Rate						
Rhythm						
Cardiac Output						
Cardiac Index *						
Left Ventricular Work						
Left Ventricular Stroke Work						
Peripheral Resistance						
AO_2 Sat.						
VO_2 Sat.						
Sat. diff.						
Fick Method C. O**						

Age _____   Weight _____   Height _____

* Cardiac Index = divide output by Body Surface area
**See page 30

SYSTEM OF CARDIOVASCULAR MONITORING AND REACTION
ON BASIS OF FICK METHOD CARDIAC OUTPUT DETERMINATIONS***

I. The Variables:

1. pulmonary artery oxygen saturation

2. radial artery or brachial artery oxygen saturation

3. pulmonary artery diastolic pressure if within 3 mm. of Hg. of wedge pressure

4. vena caval oxygen saturation (from C. V. P.)

5. Fick cardiac output
    Cardiac output=

$$\frac{3.5* \text{ x Pt's wt in kilo}}{10 \text{ x } 1.34** \text{ x Hb x (Sat \% arterial-Sat \% PA vena caval } O_2 \text{ Sat}}$$

6. thermodilution cardiac output

7. heart work

8. peripheral resistance

9. mean blood pressure - via transducer

10. hemoglobin

Constants used in formula:

*3. 5cc of oxygen per kilo is usual oxygen consumption.

**1. 34cc of oxygen is usual amount of oxygen carried by gram of hemoglobin.

***If you do outputs by both Fick and thermodilution when you do not have your thermodilution operative (breakdown of machine - it happens - or loss of pulmonary artery catheter), you then can do accurate outputs on basis of oxygen consumption from arterial and vena caval blood gases.

Flow sheet - To determine relationships of cardiac output determined by
thermodilutions and Fick method - See page 30 for directions.

Date or time:

Pulmonary artery O_2 Sat											
Radial artery O_2 Sat											
Venal caval O_2 Sat											
Cardiac Output based on Pul. artery O_2 Sat											
Cardiac Output based on vena caval O_2 Sat											
Cardiac Output based on thermodilution											
Peripheral resistance (thermodilution)											
- Cardiac Work -											
Hemoglobin											
Blood volume mg/kilo											
Weight											

Nomogram for Calculating the
Body Surface Area of Adults*

* From the formula of DuBois and DuBois, *Arch. Intern. Med.*, **17**,863 (1916): $S = W^{0.425} \times H^{0.725} \times 71.84$, or $\log S = 0.425 \log W + 0.725 \log H + 1.8564$, where S = body surface area in square centimeters, W = weight in kilograms, H = height in centimeters.

Nomogram for Calculating the
Body Surface Area of Children*

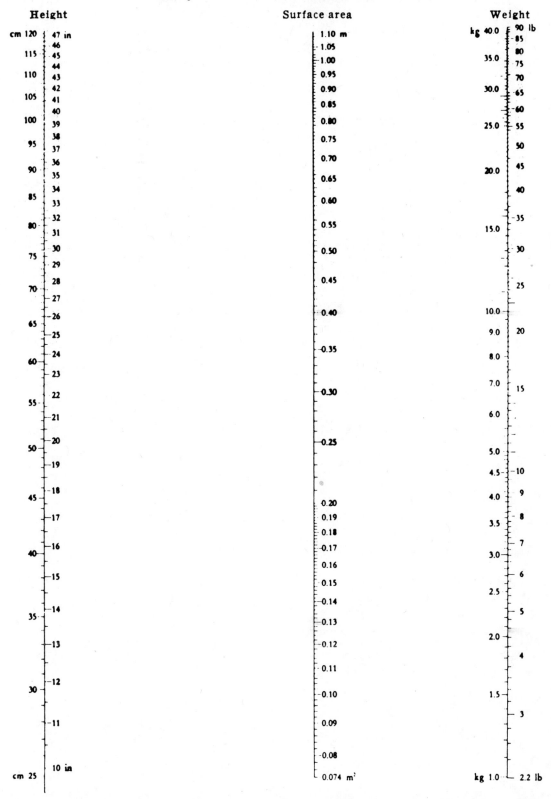

*From the formula of DuBois and DuBois, *Arch. Intern. Med.*, **17**,863 (1916):
$S = W^{0.425} \times H^{0.725} \times 71.84$, or log $S = 0.425$ log $W + 0.725$ log $H + 1.8564$,
where $S =$ body surface area in square centimeters, $W =$ weight in kilograms,
$H =$ height in centimeters.

NOTES

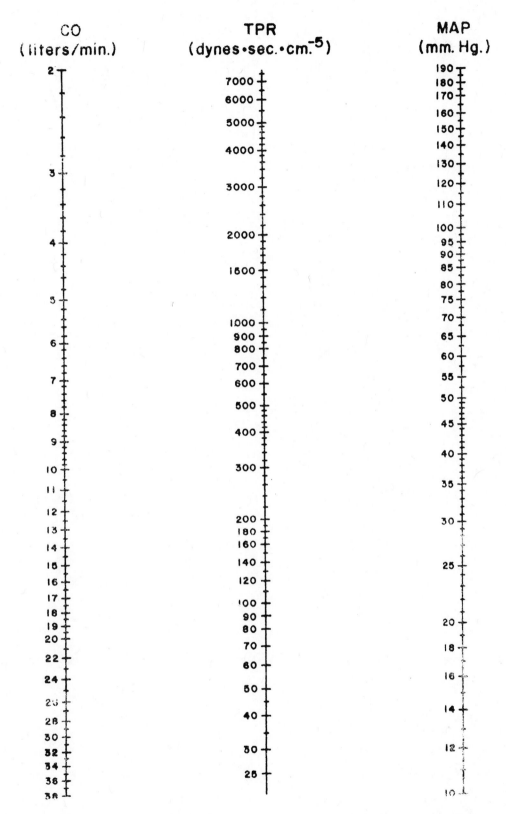

Nomogram for obtaining total peripheral resistance (TPR) from cardiac output (CO) and mean arterial pressure (MAP).

NOTES

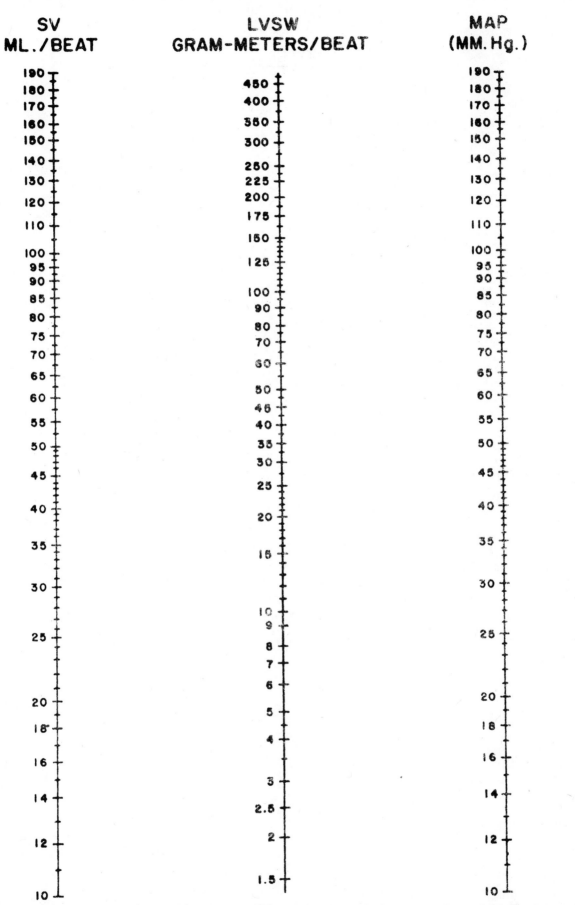

SV ML./BEAT	LVSW GRAM-METERS/BEAT	MAP (MM. Hg.)

Nomogram for obtaining left ventricular stroke work (LVSW) from stroke volumes (SV) and mean arterial pressure (MAP). An index for left ventricular stroke work may be calculated either by substituting cardiac index (CI) for cardiac output (CO) or by dividing left ventricular stroke work (LVSP) by body surface area (BSA).

NOTES

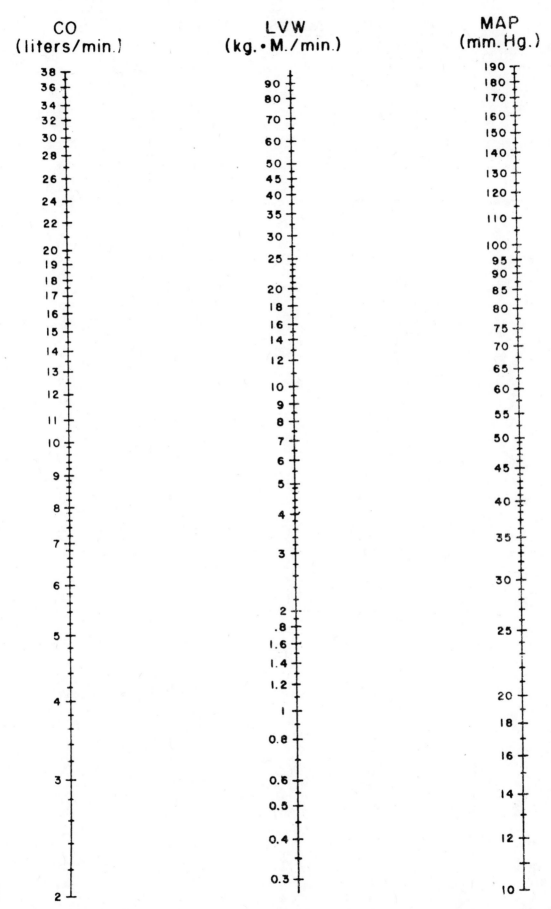

Nomogram for obtaining left ventricular work (LVW) from cardiac output (CO) and mean arterial pressure (MAP).

NOTES

SUSPECTED CORONARY FLOWSHEET

	Normal * Range	Peak Time	Day 1 12-24	Day 2	Day 3	Day 4	Day 5	Day 6	Day 7
EKG changes + or -									
Depth of Q waves									
Enzymes** LDH		3--6 days							
SGOT		18--36 hr.							
CPK									
Blood pressure***									
Cardiac rhythm****									
Isoenzymes -									
LDH$_1$ (cardiac)									
LDH$_5$ (muscle)									
CPKMB (heart)	2 ± 1								
WBC									
sed rate									

*Obtain normal and ranges from your own clinical laboratory.

**If enzyme abnormal -- automatically do isoenzymes.

***If under 90 see page 176 for Cardiac Shock System and start Cardiac Function Flowsheet.

****Cardiac rhythm -- if abnormal see pages 212-219 (EKG System.)

NOTES

BLEEDING DIATHESIS FLOWSHEET

Name					
Date					
Hospital day					
Test	Normal Labs*				
History of previous bleeding	Yes or				
Bleeding from multiple sites	No				
Platelet count					
Bleeding time					
Prothrombin time					
Partial thromboplastin time					
Thrombin time					
Blood smear for red cell fragments, platelets					
Clot solubility test					

See Bleeding Diathesis System
page 204

* Have your own laboratory fill these in.

NOTES

HYPERALIMENTATION FLOWSHEET

Name						
Date						
Hospital Day						
Value	Contingency Order Level	Page				
Weight						
Intake						
Output						
Fluid Balance	± 4					
ml. & type of hyper- alimentation						
ml. of intralipid						
Blood sugar	all readings					
Hemoglobin	<10					
Hematocrit						
WBC	>10,000					
BUN	>30					
Serum NH_4	>30					
Serum osmolality	>350					
Na	>150					
K	>5 <4					
Triglycerides	↑ 50					
Magnesium	<1.4 >1.9					
Zinc	<1					
Calcium	>10 <6					

ADDITIONS TO HYPERALIMENTATION SYSTEM
AS DETERMINED BY YOUR SERVICE

HEMODIALYSIS FLOWSHEET

Date Value	Range page	Pre-	Post-	Pre-	Post-	Pre-	Post-	Pre-	Post-	Pre-	Post-
Fluid	page										
Blood flow	200-600										
Pressure on outflow line	20-200										
Bath temperature	36°-38°										
Dialysate flow rate	200-1000										
Hours of dialysis											
Weight											
BUN	20										
Na	140-150										
K											
pH											
HCO$_3$											
Base excess acid											
Hemoglobin											
Hematocrit											
Platelets											
WBC											
Reticulocyte count											
Stabs											
PCO$_2$											
PO$_2$											
% Sat. O$_2$											
Phosphorus											
Glucose											
Uric acid											
Cholesterol											
Total protein											
Bilirubin											
Alkaline phosphatase											
SGOT											
Chloride											
Calcium	4-8										

See Dialysis System page 163

NOTES

IMMUNODEPRESSED OR CANCER CHEMOTHERAPY FLOWSHEET

Hospital day										
Value										
WBC										
% Polyps										
% Eosinophiles										
% Lymphocytes										
Platelets										
Hemoglobin										
Reticulocytes										
Gamma A										
Gamma G										
Total complement										
C^3										
Skin test - mumps										
SK-SD										
Candida										
PPD										
T-cell %										
PHA response										
M.I.F. *										
N.B.T. **										
Other tests										
Therapy:										

See Compromised Host System - page 205

* Macrophage Inhibition Factor

** Nitro Blue Tetrazolium

NOTES

MODIFICATIONS FOR AGE

AGE OVER 60: As a general rule patients over 60 do not tolerate sodium well, and unless there is definite evidence of hyponatremia (level under 120) they do better if they have no more than 2 liters of saline or Ringer's lactate (18 gm. of salt) per day -- and preferably <u>less</u>.

Renal excretion of antibiotics is definitely impaired after age 60 and that is why our antibiotic orders (see Antibiotic Fail-Safe System) are adjusted for age.

Patients over 60 tolerate barbiturates poorly and, when possible, other sedatives such as chloral hydrate should be used, or use only 1/2 dose of barbiturates.

Patients over 60 are approaching the last third of their life span, often with many rickety organ systems, therefore they must be treated with the extra attention befitting their age; <u>their right to die must be respected with particular care,</u> and every effort must be made to keep them in touch with their environment (night lights, etc.) and their loved ones.

AGE UNDER 10: I personally believe seriously ill children should be in a Children's Critical Care area because I, as an internist, have finally come to the conclusion that they are NOT small adults. They are children and must be cared for as such.

Seriously ill children should always have subclavian lines.

Their parents must be able to sit at their bedsides at all times (if the parents can stand it).

On a relative basis, children need higher dosages per weight of digoxin, fluids, and antibiotics than do adults.

Children usually tolerate hyperalimentation without the addition of insulin to the bottle.

WEIGHT OVER 250 LBS.

(Use nomograms on pages 32 and 33 to convert to kilos.)

Obese patients are particularly prone to pulmonary complications and have a tendency to store certain drugs in their fat stores for later release. They tend to be less mobile than the usual patient (that's why they are fat) and therefore have a greater than average tendency to have embolic phenomena and phlebitis.

ACTIVE CONTINGENCY ORDERS FOR WEIGHT OVER 250 LBS. -

1. IPPB every 6 hours.

2. Keep patient as upright as possible.

3. Encourage deep breathing.

4. Encourage maximum ambulation.

WEIGHT CHANGE

ACTIVE CONTINGENCY ORDERS FOR WEIGHT GAIN OF OVER THREE POUNDS FROM PREVIOUS DAY -

1. Give edecrin, 50 mg., if weight is <u>over</u> 120 pounds OR
    give edecrin, 25 mg., if weight is <u>under</u> 120 pounds.

2. If patient does not put out 500 cc. of urine in the next 6 hours,
    give lasix, 200 mg., if weight is <u>over</u> 120 pounds OR
    give lasix, 100 mg., if weight is <u>under</u> 120 pounds.

3. If patient still does not <u>increase</u> the urinary output significantly in the next
    6 hours, SLOW rate of <u>fluid administration</u> to rate of 2000 ml. per day
    plus urine output and follow CONTINGENCY ORDERS for Urine output
    (page 55 and 57), Pulmonary Artery Pressure (page 89), and BUN (page 113).

INSENSIBLE FLUID LOSS

This represents water lost by evaporation and through the lungs. It is determined by the following simple, logical formula:

$$\left(\begin{array}{ccc}\text{Initial} & & \text{Intake}\\ \text{Weight} & \text{PLUS} & \text{in}\\ \text{in Kilos} & & \text{Kilos}\end{array}\right) \text{ MINUS } \left(\begin{array}{ccc}\text{Urine} & \text{PLUS} & \text{2nd}\\ \text{Output} & & \text{Weight}\end{array}\right) = \begin{array}{l}\text{INSENSIBLE}\\ \text{FLUID}\\ \text{LOSS}\end{array}$$

For example: First weight 70 kilos and the patient gets 6 liters of fluid = 76

Second Weight 72 kilos, patient puts out 2 liters of urine = 74

<u>The insensible fluid loss is 2 liters.</u>

A normal person loses 1500 ml. of insensible fluid per day.

A hyperventilating person loses up to 3 or 4 liters a day.

An adult burn patient being treated by the exposure method loses at the rate of the following formula for the first 14 days. *

Per Cent of Burn	Insensible Fluid Loss
4% - 19%	2400 ml.
20% - 59%	2640 ml.
60%	3840 ml.

Based on 50 consecutive patients treated at St. Mary's Burn Center.* After the first 14 days these values are reduced 50%.

ACTIVE CONTINGENCY ORDERS FOR INSENSIBLE FLUID LOSS -

The daily fluid requirements of a critically ill patient in whom fluid balance is any problem should include D/5/W, given in a volume to replace insensible fluid loss.

* B.A. Waisbren: Treatment of severe burns.
Comprehensive Therapy 2 : 33-42, January 1976.

URINE OUTPUT OVER 4000 MILLILITERS

The most common cause of a high urine output is fluid overload by I.V. fluids or excess water intake by mouth. Urine output in a normal individual should be around 1500 ml. per day on an oral intake of 2500 to 3000 ml. per day. Seriously ill patients usually get more than 3000 ml. of fluid a day and, with normal kidneys, should put out in the urine their intake minus 1500 to 2000 ml. of insensible fluid loss.

If urine output is OVER 4000 ml. per day:

DIAGNOSTIC CONTINGENCY ORDERS:
1. Check amount of I.V. fluid orders and intake by mouth.
2. Check urine and serum osmolality, blood volume, and BUN.
3. Note whether there is brain injury, oat cell carcinoma of the lung, recent severe injury to the head, a severe burn, or recent cancer chemotherapy.

DIFFERENTIAL DIAGNOSES WILL BE BETWEEN:
1. Excessive intake.
2. Diabetes insipidus -- lack of vasopressin, normal sodium, low blood volume, usually apparent intercranial problem, normal kidney function.
3. Inappropriate antidiuretic hormone -- low sodium, normal blood volume. Associated with carcinoma of lung and pancreas and severe trauma or burn. Patient psychotic.
4. Regaining of cardiac and renal compensation.
5. Tubular renal disease.
6. Excessive diuresis often caused by hyperalimentation.

ACTIVE CONTINGENCY ORDERS:
1. Slow down fluids if they are over 6000 ml. a day.
2. Stop routine orders for diuretics.
3. If serum sodium is normal and there is any indication of diabetes insipidus, try one cc. of pitressin I.M. (20 pressor units). If this stems urine flow, this diagnosis will be more seriously considered.
4. If serum sodium is low, blood volume normal, and serum osmolality in normal range (290-310) and patient has carcinoma or received cancer chemotherapy, or received a severe injury or blow, or has a brain tumor, or has a severe burn -- consider inappropriate antidiuretic hormone and restrict fluid to 1000 ml. per day.
5. If renal function studies abnormal, consider the renal tubules as the culprit and stop nephrotoxic drugs and delineate kidney disease.
6. If the patient is merely losing edema fluids or regaining cardiac compensation, be thankful that he is putting out urine well and do not let him get dehydrated.

NOTES

URINE OUTPUT LESS THAN 1000 MILLILITERS

Hourly urine outputs should be kept on all seriously ill patients (see hourly log form for this on page 25). If the output falls below 40 ml. per hour for two hours in a row--treat for incipient renal shutdown in the following manner.

DIAGNOSTIC CONTINGENCY ORDERS FOR INCIPIENT RENAL SHUTDOWN:
1. Hourly urine output
2. 6-hour creatinine clearance which also gives you the creatinine level
3. daily 24-hour excretion of Na and K and protein
4. Urinalysis STAT with special request for search for renal failure casts
5. Blood culture
6. CBC
7. Arterial blood gases
8. Blood pressure
9. Urine sodium concentration

ACTIVE CONTINGENCY ORDERS FOR IMPENDING RENAL SHUTDOWN:
1. STOP all drugs that may be nephrotoxic. Most common offenders are kanamycin, gentamicin, polymyxin B, streptomycin, methicillin, and trobicin.
2. Give fluid load in the next hour--one liter of D/5/W--BUT SLOW THIS IF:
   a. The mean pulmonary artery pressure rises more than 5.
   b. The pulse increases over 25 beats per minute from previous rate.
   c. The CVP goes over 15.
   d. The jugular veins distend.
   e. The patient coughs up frothy sputum.
   f. The patient becomes excessively short of breath.
3. Give either edecrin, 50 mg., or lasix, 80 mg., intravenously. If, in the first hour, this does not cause diuresis--give the lasix if you have already given the edecrin or vice versa.
4. After the fluid load and diuretic, give $12\frac{1}{2}$ gm. of mannitol in the next 500 ml. of fluid that you are running in. If this does not start urine output, give decadron, 50 mg. in 300 ml. of fluid I.V.
5. If moderate diuretic dose does not work, give lasix, 15 mg. (Check WBC for next 5 days for depression of it, due to lasix, which is rare).
6. If, after these maneuvers, urine output is still below 200 ml. per hour, adjust fluid intake to 2000 ml. per day and stop all K-containing fluids.
7. Check K levels every 12 hours and, if over 5.5, give Kayexalate, 30 gm., either rectally or by stomach tube, every 6 hours.
8. If K is above 6, dialyze, either by hemo- or peritoneal dialysis (page 163)

NOTES

POSITIVE FLUID BALANCE GREATER THAN 4000 MILLILITERS PER 24 HOURS

The patient should be in essential fluid balance, i.e., intake should equal output. If balance is over 4000 ml., the patient has either heart failure, kidney failure, fluid overload, or is holding fluid.

DIAGNOSTIC CONTINGENCY ORDERS FOR FLUID BALANCE GREATER THAN 4000 MILLILITERS:
1. Check fluid orders to see whether oral intake plus the running I.V. orders are not resulting in fluid overload.
2. Check blood volume and follow CONTINGENCY ORDERS in its regard (pages 78-79).
3. Check CVP, pulmonary artery pressure, listen for gallop rhythm, look for distended neck veins, get chest x-ray and EKG (pages 212-219).
4. Get renal function studies, creatinine clearance, BUN, urinalysis, serum albumins and globulins.

ACTIVE CONTINGENCY ORDERS FOR FLUID BALANCE GREATER THAN 4000 MILLILITERS:
1. Reduce fluid intake to 2000 ml. over insensible fluid loss.
2. If blood volume is over 70 ml/kilo give edecrin, 50 mg.
3. If studies obtained under Diagnostic Order 3 indicate heart failure--digitalize with Digitalis System on page 196.
4. If renal function studies are abnormal, hold nephrotoxic drugs (page 194).

FLUID BALANCE NEGATIVE 4000 MILLILITERS

If fluid balance is less than 4000 ml., the patient is putting out four more liters of fluid than he is taking in.

DIAGNOSTIC CONTINGENCY ORDERS FOR FLUID BALANCE LESS THAN 4000 MILLILITERS:
1. Check loss through nasogastric tube and/or get a flat plate of the abdomen -- you may have a high bowel obstruction.
2. If large loss is from diarrhea, get stool culture, smear of stool for Staphylococcus, and flat plate of abdomen. You may be seeing acute enterocolitis, secondary to antibiotics use in serious illness.

ACTIVE CONTINGENCY ORDERS FOR FLUID BALANCE NEGATIVE 4000 MILILITERS:
1. If urine output is greater than 4000 ml. follow program on page 55.

ARTERIAL OXYGEN TENSION OF UNDER 70 MEANS THERE IS NOT ENOUGH
AVAILABLE OXYGEN IN THE RED BLOOD CELLS TO KEEP THE BODY'S CELLS
ADEQUATELY SUPPLIED--THIS MUST ALWAYS BE ATTENDED TO:

POSSIBLE REASONS FOR PaO_2 OF LESS THAN 70:
1. Some patients with chronic lung disease have adapted to this level of PaO_2 so a history of emphysema or chronic bronchitis and long-standing lung problems can lessen some of your concern.
2. Obstruction in the pharynx or bronchi or damage to the alveolar cells themselves can cause this so your diagnostic and therapeutic efforts must be determined by, and directed toward, the cause of the problem.
3. Lab technician might have tested venous blood.
4. The patient might not be breathing deeply enough.

DIAGNOSTIC CONTINGENCY ORDERS FOR PaO_2 UNDER 70:
1. Chest x-ray
2. If chest x-ray is negative get lung scan with xenon washout
3. LDH with isoenzymes
4. EKG
5. Get blood gases before and after 100% O_2 given by mask
6. Check for heart failure, distended veins, frothy sputum, tachycardia, and rales
7. Check nasopharynx and throat for obstruction and secretions
8. Listen for obstruction and secretion

ACTIVE CONTINGENCY ORDERS FOR PaO_2 UNDER 70:
1. Do a vigorous tracheal toilet and encourage more active respiration.
2. STOP sedation.
3. Get an opinion regarding fiberoptic bronchoscopy.
4. Start O_2 --8 liters a minute with a 40% venturi type mask (IF PATIENT DOES NOT HAVE CHRONIC EMPHYSEMA).
5. Notify M.D. as to the finding.
6. If PaO_2 is under 50, after doing above 1, 2, 3, and 4, prepare to start assisted respiration with a respirator (page 157).
7. If patient has chronic emphysema make decisions on basis of pCO_2 (page 63, 67) and clinical status.

NOTES

IF THE $PaCO_2$ IS UNDER 25, THE MOST COMMON REASON IS HYPERVENTILATION CAUSED BY ANXIETY -- BUT

If it is NOT this, the $PaCO_2$ is low due to the body's attempt to keep the 1:20 ratio by blowing off CO_2 as the $NaHCO_2$ is being neutralized by acids being abnormally produced--but not excreted--by the body.

DIAGNOSTIC CONTINGENCY ORDERS WHEN THE $PaCO_2$ IS UNDER 25:
1. BUN and/creatinine--if they are elevated, you have the explanation, i.e., inability of the kidneys to excrete acid by-products of cell metabolism. Get renal function studies (page 113).
2. Fasting blood sugar (pages 133-135). Diabetic acidosis is a common cause of a low CO_2 because of fatty acids produced when carbohydrate is not being burned for lack of insulin.
3. Salicylate level--aspirin ingestion is common cause of a low CO_2 due to acid products released by cell damage due to the aspirin.
4. Drug intoxication panel, which should include levels of methadone, amphetamine, cocaine, pentobarbital, phenobarbital, glutethimide, meprobamate, quinine, and phenothiazines.
5. Lactic acid level elevation means cells are not metabolizing aerobically (page 68).

ACTIVE CONTINGENCY ORDERS WHEN THE $PaCO_2$ IS UNDER 25:
1. If blood sugar level is over 300, institute following DIABETIC COMA PROGRAM.
   a. Check urine for acetone.
   b. Do serial serum assay for acetone.
   c. Give insulin by following this schedule:

   Blood sugar over 500 - 100 units regular insulin I.V. - check every 2 hours

   Blood sugar 400 - 499 - 60 units regular insulin I.V. - check every 2 hours

   Blood sugar 300 - 399 - 50 units regular insulin I.V. - check every 2 hours

   Blood sugar 200 - 299 - 20 units regular insulin I.V. - check every 2 hours

2. If salicylate level over 40:
   a. Give 2 ampules of $NaHCO_3$ (44.6 mEq per ampule) each hour the pH is under 7.3 for five hours. Or use formula - pt. weight in kg. x 0.3 x base deficit = total mEq. of NaH as minims of NaH carb.
   b. Give saline at rate to get urine output above 100 ml. if patient's age is under 50. This can start at one liter an hour for five hours.
   c. Institute a close watch for respiratory difficulties and need for respirator.
   d. Consider hemodialysis (page 163).

3. If BUN is over 35 follow UREMIA PROGRAM:
    a. Get urea clearance, urinalysis, 24-hour urine for albumin, and hourly urine outputs.
    b. Treat the underlying renal disease.
    c. Consider dialysis (page 163).
    d. Put on 40 gm. protein dietary intake program.

4. If BUN, FBS, and drug levels are normal, hyperventilation is the most common cause of low $PaCO_2$.
    a. Give Valium, 10 mg. by mouth every 8 hours.
    b. Reassure patient and arrange for family visits, etc.

ARTERIAL PaCO$_2$ GREATER THAN 45

If the PaCO$_2$ is over 45 the patient is not ridding the lungs of CO$_2$, either due to oversedation, weakness, chest injury, or too much dead space. The elevated PaCO$_2$ causes his red cells to hold on to O$_2$, thus denying it to his other cells. As the PaCO$_2$ is lowered by assisted ventilation, potassium tends to return to cells so K levels must be monitored very carefully as this is done.

DIAGNOSTIC CONTINGENCY ORDERS:

1. If patient has chronic lung disease, has a normal pH, and is comfortable and alert, the PaCO$_2$ may be normal for him - so do nothing.

2. Draw barbiturate and any other sedative drug levels available to you.

3. Get chest x-ray and ask that special attention be paid to possibility of broken ribs and/or pulmonary emphysema.

4. Get potassium levels every 4 hours as you correct the PaCO$_2$, especially if the patient is receiving digitalis, and follow CONTINGENCY ORDERS for K (page 127).

ACTIVE CONTINGENCY ORDERS:

1. Give naloxine (Narcan), 4 mg. I.V., if the patient has been on morphine, codeine, demerol, or any other narcotic and is not suffering from chronic lung disease. If you do not know for sure - give Narcan as therapeutic test. (in patients brought in from the emergency room)

2. Encourage deep breathing by IPPB every hour for 10 minutes until CO$_2$ goes to under 40 and continue this at rate to keep it there.

3. Examine nasopharynx and suction to relieve ball valve type obstruction.

4. If there are broken ribs, use rib splint and morphine sulfate, gr. 1/6, so he can breathe without too much pain.

5. If you cannot encourage voluntary breathing enough to get the PCO$_2$ under 50 within several hours, arrange for the respirator--it will be necessary (page 157).

HCO$_3$ -- BICARBONATE BELOW 22

Bicarbonate below 22 usually indicates a metabolic acidosis and it is compensatory for carbonic acid being pushed out of the system by inorganic acids.

DIAGNOSTIC CONTINGENCY ORDERS FOR HCO$_3$, BELOW 22:

Follow Contingency orders for pH, (page 71), BUN (pages 113, 115), and lactic acid (page 68).

ACTIVE CONTINGENCY ORDERS FOR HCO$_3$ BELOW 22:

1. NaHCO$_3$ should be given hourly until HCO$_3$ is above 14 in diabetic acidosis (Diabetic Coma System, page 209).

2. In other situations for HCO$_3$ will usually correct itself as a result of the reactions indicated for other abnormalities of acid base.

HCO$_3$ -- BICARBONATE ABOVE 28

Bicarbonate is regulated by the kidney tubules, which exchange hydrogen ions for bicarbonate in the proximal tubules. This mechanism works to keep twenty times as much HCO$_3$ in the serum as CO$_2$, which is the fundamental buffering mechanism of the body.

DIAGNOSTIC AND ACTIVE CONTINGENCY ORDERS FOR HCO$_3$ ABOVE 28:
1. Check pH -- if within normal range, do not treat until diagnosis is established. It may be quite normal for the patient to have elevated HCO$_3$.

2. Check potassium level and blood volume and follow CONTINGENCY ORDERS written for them (page 127). Persistent HCO$_3$ elevation in the presence of normal kidneys is a good clue to intracellular K deficiency, so elevate K level to 4.5 by adjusting schedule shown on page 127 up 25%. (The most common cause of HCO$_3$ above 28 is K loss due to diuretics.)

3. HCO$_3$ may be elevated as a compensatory mechanism for CO$_2$ retention so follow CONTINGENCIES for CO$_2$ above 40 (page 63, 65).

4. HCO$_3$ may be elevated because of NaHCO$_3$ administration. If this is the situation and the pH is still low, discontinue the NaHCO$_3$.

LACTIC ACID GREATER THAN 2.8

An elevated lactic acid is always a very poor prognostic sign. It means that the body's cells are not able to oxidize pyruvic acid to CO_2 and water and must use the anaerobic route that results in the production of lactic acid. The lactic acid per se does not kill the patient, it is merely the sign that the cells are not working correctly. A lactic acid above 5 almost always means impending death. The most common cause of lactic acidosis now is the oral hypoglycemic agent phenformin (DBI) but it is a frequent terminal finding in burns and gram-negative shock.

ACTIVE CONTINGENCY ORDERS FOR LACTIC ACID OVER 2.8:

1. Attempt to get PO_2 above 100, using hyperbaric O_2 if necessary.

2. Attempt urine output of over 200 ml. per hour by diuretics and increasing fluid intake.

3. Treat infections to the maximum.

4. Consider dialysis if phenformin is the cause or if there is not a salutary trend.

5. Give regular insulin at rate to get blood sugar to level under 200.

6. Digitalize and normalize cardiac output.

7. Give methylene blue, 200 mg. I.V. every 6 hours. This acts as an intracellular hydrogen ion receptor and, while not proven, is worthwhile trying due to the terrible prognosis of this condition. (Oliva, Am. J. Med., Feb., 1970)

BASIC EXCESS GREATER THAN 3

This value summarizes the state of the buffering system by determining its effect on O_2 dissociation by red blood cells. The more alkaline the blood, the more the cells hold on to oxygen.

If the base excess is over 3 and going up, this is a good indication of metabolic alkalosis and it indicates that you should go easy on the injection of $NaHCO_3$.

DIAGNOSTIC AND ACTIVE CONTINGENCY ORDERS FOR BASE EXCESS OVER 3:
1. Discontinue $NaHCO_3$

2. Follow CONTINGENCY ORDERS for remainder of blood gas determinations (pages 61-73).

ACID EXCESS (BASE DEFICIT)

Why there is an acceptance of the terrible term negative base excess is hard to understand and I hope all of you will be able to convince your laboratories to report it as acid excess instead. This value is, for all intents and purposes, an indicator of metabolic acidosis, which is caused by kidney failure, diabetic acidosis, or cell failure (lactic acidosis). (Page 68).

DIAGNOSTIC AND ACTIVE CONTINGENCY ORDERS FOR NEGATIVE BASE EXCESS OVER 3 (i.e., AN ACID EXCESS):
1. Follow remainder of CONTINGENCY ORDERS indicated by the blood gases.

2. Order BUN, lactic acid, blood sugar, blood pH, salicylate level, and poison screen panel of your hospital.

ARTERIAL O_2 SATURATION MINUS VENOUS O_2 SATURATION *
-- INCREASE OF 10 IN THE DIFFERENCE

When the venous O_2 saturation is declining more rapidly than the arterial O_2 the flow of blood is slowing and more O_2 is getting extracted from the red blood cells on the venous side. Thus the AO_2 saturation--VO_2 saturation constitutes a "poor man's cardiac output".

DIAGNOSTIC CONTINGENCY ORDERS WHEN AO_2 SATURATION MINUS VO_2 SATURATION IS INCREASING:
1. Get serial cardiac outputs if available

2. Check pulmonary artery and wedge pressures and follow CONTINGENCY ORDERS indicated by them.

3. Get chest x-ray for pulmonary edema.

4. If pulmonary artery pressures are not available, get CVP and follow orders indicated. Repeat blood gases hourly until it is reversed.

ACTIVE CONTINGENCY ORDERS WHEN AO_2 SATURATION MINUS VO_2 SATURATION IS INCREASING:
1. Digitalis by the Digitalis System (page 196).

2. Slow fluids to 50 ml/hour until CVP or pulmonary artery pressure is normal.

3. If blood volume is normal or elevated, give edecrin, 50 mg. I.V.

4. If there is a bradycardia this is an indication of the need for atropine and then, possibly, pacing.

---

* The closer to the pulmonary artery the venous blood is drawn the better, and the more helpful the AO_2 - VO_2 difference will be. Usually the CVP line is the most available site to draw the venous blood.

pH BELOW 7.3

The pH represents the acidity of the body fluids. The lower it is, the more acid is the body. A pH of under 7.3 is <u>always</u> a serious matter which must be explained and treated. It gets into abnormal ranges when the body's buffer system can no longer maintain proper ratios of acid and base. The cause of low pH is abnormal acidity because:

1. CO_2 acid is not being blown off by the lungs and disposed of as CO_2.

2. The body is producing too much acid because of abnormal metabolism of cells--either due to lack of insulin or cell damage.

3. The kidneys are unable to excrete normal acid products--uremic acidosis.

Therefore, acidosis can be caused by abnormalities in the lungs, kidneys, or cells.

DIAGNOSTIC CONTINGENCY ORDERS FOR pH BELOW 7.3:
1. Get complete blood gases, lactic acid, salicylic level, blood sugar, chest x-ray, BUN, and serum acetone level.

   If $PaCO_2$ is elevated--you have lung acidosis.
   If $PaCO_2$ is depressed--you have kidney acidosis.
   If lactic acid, acetone, or salicylate level is elevated--you have cellular acidosis.

ACTIVE CONTINGENCY ORDERS FOR pH BELOW 7.3:
1. Monitor EKG and follow CONTINGENCY ORDERS for arrhythmia (page 212)

2. If pH down and CO_2 up:

   a. Encourage deep breathing
   b. IPPB every hour for 10 minutes
   c. Follow CO_2 orders on page 63, 65
   d. If there are broken ribs, use rib splint and morphine, gr. 1/6, every four hours
   e. If you cannot get pCO_2 under 50 and the patient is not a chronic respiratory failure victim, prepare for respirator and/or fiberoptic bronchoscopy.

3. If pH down, CO_2 down, and BUN up--follow Renal Failure program (page 113, 57).

4. If pH down, CO_2 down, and ketones up--follow Diabetic Coma program (page 209).

5. If pH down, CO_2 down, and lactic acid up--follow Lactic Acidosis program (page 209).

6. If pH down, CO_2 down, and salicylate level up--follow this program for Salicylate Poisoning:

   a. Place indwelling catheter
   b. Saline at 1000 ml. an hour to get maximum urine output
   c. Monitor EKG
   d. NaHCarbonate, 44 mEq. (one ampule) every 15 minutes until pH above 7.3 or bicarbonate level above 28
   e. If these measures do not cause diuresis, consider hemodialysis or exchange transfusion unless patient is improving.

PaO$_2$ WITH 100% OXYGEN BY MASK:

DECREASE OF 10 FROM PREVIOUS READING

A lowering of the extent to which 100% O$_2$ can raise the PaO$_2$ means that an increasing number of alveoli are not transporting oxygen to the red cells that are passing them by (increasing shunt). Thus, if the PaO$_2$ shows a decreasing reaction to breathing, 100% oxygen by mouth is indicated. When the PaO$_2$ is less than 55 while the patient is on 100% oxygen, positive action must be taken or the patient probably will die.

DIAGNOSTIC CONTINGENCY ORDERS WITH INCREASING SHUNT:
1. Chest x-ray

2. Sputum culture

3. Cardiac output (page 28).

4. Simultaneous arterial and venous oxygen saturation at 4-hour intervals (page 29, 70).

5. Repeat tests after IPPB treatment and maximum efforts to clear trachea and lungs.

ACTIVE CONTINGENCY ORDERS WITH INCREASING SHUNT:
1. If PaO$_2$ is under 55 on 100% oxygen, give edecrin, 50 mg., and digitalize the patient (page 196).

2. Use maximum efforts to clear tracheobronchial tree.

3. Decrease sedation and give Nalixin, 10 mg., if patient had been on morphine or its derivatives.

4. Add PEEP or CPAP to respirator if patient is on one.

NOTES

To assess a shunt . . .

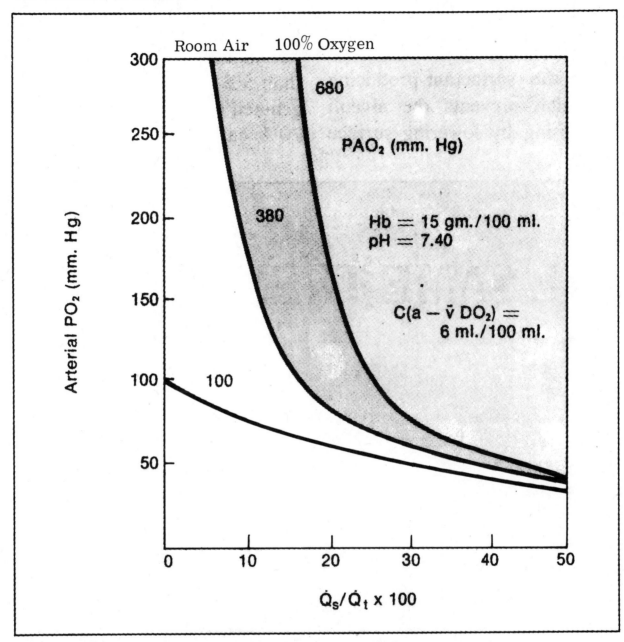

If your patient's arterial PO₂ has dropped below 65 mm. Hg, this
nomogram will help quantify the degree of shunting in his pulmonary
circulation by giving the gradient between the PO₂ of inspired gas and
arterial blood. Alveolar PO₂ will be close to 680 mm. Hg if the
patient breathes 100% oxygen for 15 minutes. Then measure arterial PO₂,
follow the appropriate ordinate across to the 680 alveolar PO₂ curve, and
carry it down to the percent pulmonary shunt ($\dot{Q}_s/\dot{Q}_t$). Thus a patient
who responds to pure oxygen with an arterial PO₂ of 180 has a danger-level
20% shunt with a gradient of 500. On room air, alveolar PO₂ is 100
and the same shunt gives an arterial PO₂ of 60 and a gradient of 40.

NOTES

TIDAL VOLUME BELOW 500

This is determined by a simple flowmeter which is placed in the mouth or over the opening of the tracheostomy tube. If the patient cannot move more than 500 cc. of air per breath, he will go into respiratory failure, so attention must be given immediately to the problem. In actuality the tidal volume is most helpful as one of the determinants of when a patient may be taken off the respirator. If the blood gases are o.k., it is not a value that causes anxiety per se.

DIAGNOSTIC CONTINGENCY ORDERS FOR TIDAL VOLUME UNDER 500:
1. Get arterial blood gases.

2. Get chest x-ray.

3. Check for broken ribs or chest injury.

4. Check for central nervous system depression, either due to drugs or a CVA.

5. Check stability of chest if recent thoracotomy or crush injury.

ACTIVE CONTINGENCY ORDERS FOR TIDAL VOLUME BELOW 500:
1. Encourage deep breathing.

2. Discontinue sedation if this is the problem.

3. Put on rib splint and give morphine, gr. 1/6, for pain relief if broken ribs are the problem.

4. Put sand bags to immobilize one side of chest if instability is the problem. (Do this under the direction of the attending physician.) Actually, you probably will want to stabilize the chest by machine assisted ventilation, since sand bags are a bit old-fashioned.

BLOOD VOLUME GREATER THAN 75 ML/KILO

This is a very accurate value determined by injecting radioactive chromate into the blood stream and measuring its dilution at a set time. The more diluted it is, the greater the blood volume. This test will give false results in the presence of active bleeding, in which case it will give a falsely large volume.

There is a wide range of normal in blood volumes--55 ml/kilo to 75 ml/kilo--but day by day changes in blood volume are very helpful in that they compare each day's volume with that of the day before.

DIAGNOSTIC CONTINGENCY ORDERS FOR BLOOD VOLUME GREATER THAN 75 ML/KILO:
1. If the blood volume is over 75 ml/kilo, the patient is probably overloaded with fluids.
   a. Check weight daily
   b. Have patient on measured intake and output

ACTIVE CONTINGENCY ORDERS FOR BLOOD VOLUME GREATER THAN 75 ML/KILO:
1. Give edecrin, 50 mg. I.V.--if weight over 150 lbs.
   Give edecrin, 30 mg. I.V.--if weight 120-150 lbs.

OR

Give lasix, 40 mg. I.V.--if weight over 150 lbs.
Give edecrin, 30 mg. I.V.--if weight 120--150 lbs.

(If there is ANY question of liver disease, give the lasix rather than the edecrin.)

2. If blood pressure is over 100 and urine output over 35 ml/hour, slow fluids to a maximum of 75 ml/hour.

BLOOD VOLUME LESS THAN 45 ML/KILO

When blood volume is less than 45 ml/kilo, your patient is hypovolemic. The rate of correction will depend on his clinical condition and age. Rule of thumb states "older the patient, more gently is volume replacement mounted".

DIAGNOSTIC CONTINGENCY ORDERS FOR BLOOD VOLUME LESS THAN
45 ML/KILO:
1. Check for bleeding.

2. Do rectal and look for tarry stool.

3. Check BUN -- if it has been rising in face of good urine output, the patient probably has G.I. bleeding.

ACTIVE CONTINGENCY ORDERS FOR BLOOD VOLUME LESS THAN
45 ML/KILO:
1. If blood pressure is below 100, give plasmanate, saline, or D/5/W at 250 ml. per hour until CVP is over one or pulmonary artery pressure is over 8.

2. If hemoglobin is under 11, give 500 cc. of whole blood.

3. If hemoglobin is under 9, give 1000 cc. of whole blood.

NOTES

BLOOD PRESSURE UNDER 90

Of all the indications of clinical trouble I consider a fall in blood pressure below 90 the most important; and below 50 means death unless something is done. Of particular importance is the fact that some patients with gram-negative and cardiogenic shock clinically look well, with blood pressures of under 50 almost to the moment of their death. So--hypotension must always be reacted to with alarm and alacrity.

DIAGNOSTIC CONTINGENCY ORDERS FOR BLOOD PRESSURE UNDER 90:

1. Get blood volume, CBC, and check for bleeding to rule out hypovolemic shock.

2. Get blood culture, CBC, temperature, chest x-ray, urine culture for gram-negative shock.

3. Get flat plate of abdomen, serum amylase, abdominal ultrasound for abdominal catastrophic shock.

4. Get EKG, CPK, LDH, pulmonary artery pressure for cardiogenic shock and for complete heart block.

5. Get blood gases for anoxemic shock.

6. Do neurological exam and lumbar puncture for CNS cause of shock.

7. Get drug ingestion panel and blood gases for metabolic or drug-induced shock.

8. Get blood gases, check x-ray and pulmonary angiogram, and order LDH with isoenzymes for pulmonary embolus.

ACTIVE CONTINGENCY ORDERS FOR BLOOD PRESSURE BELOW 90:
1. Follow the algorithm on page 83.

NOTES

ALGORITHM FOR SUDDEN HYPOTENSION

DO COMPLETE HISTORY AND PHYSICAL - THIS WILL USUALLY DISTINGUISH
CAUSE.

IF CORONARY

GET: EKG CPK PULMONARY ARTERY PRESSURE	USE CARDIOGENIC SHOCK SYSTEM PAGE 176

IF NOT CORONARY OCCLUSION

GET: CBC BLOOD VOLUME PRESSURE CHECK FOR: BLEEDING PULMONARY ARTERY PRESSURE	IF HYPOVOLEMIC--USE HYPOVOLEMIC SHOCK SYSTEM. PAGE 173

IF NOT HYPOVOLEMIA

IF: STAB COUNT OVER 50 TEMPERATURE OVER 101° NO OTHER OBVIOUS CAUSE OF SHOCK GET: BLOOD CULTURE	USE GRAM- NEGATIVE SHOCK SYSTEM. PAGE 174

IF NOT GRAM-NEGATIVE SHOCK

IF: EKG SHOWS RIGHT AXIS PaO_2 IS DOWN LUNG SCAN IS POSITIVE INORDINATELY DYSPNEIC	TREAT FOR PULMONARY EMBOLUS SYSTEM. PAGE 189

IF NOT PULMONARY EMBOLUS

IF: PATIENT HAS JUST RECEIVED A DRUG INJECTION THERE IS UNUSUAL SHORTNESS OF BREATH THERE IS A HISTORY OF PENICILLIN OR ASPIRIN SHOCK	USE ANAPHY- LACTIC SHOCK SYSTEM. PAGE 180

IF NOT ANAPHYLACTIC

IF: SHOCK STILL UNEXPLAINED -- DRAW CORTISOL LEVEL	GIVE 20 MG. DECADRON FOR POSSIBLE ADRENAL INSUFFICIENCY.

IF STILL NOT EXPLAINED

START ALL OVER WITH HISTORY AND PHYSICAL EXAMINATION AND FIGURE
IT OUT BEFORE THE PATIENT DIES! - GETTING AS MUCH CONSULTATION
AS NECESSARY.

NOTES

BLOOD PRESSURE OVER 250 -- SUDDEN RISE OF OVER 100 -- OR DIASTOLIC PRESSURE OVER 140

DIAGNOSTIC CONTINGENCY ORDERS FOR BLOOD PRESSURE OVER 250-- SUDDEN RISE OF OVER 100--OR DIASTOLIC PRESSURE OVER 140:

1. Check neurological for a stroke or brain tumor.

2. 24-hour urines for catecholamines or other screening test for pheochromocytoma.

3. Monitor EKG and follow CONTINGENCY ORDERS

ACTIVE CONTINGENCY ORDERS FOR BLOOD PRESSURE OVER 250--SUDDEN RISE OF OVER 100--OR DIASTOLIC PRESSURE OVER 140:

1. Diazoxide, 300 mg. I.V. bolus--may repeat every 4 hours--

<u>or alternatively</u>

1a. Nitroprusside, 50 mg. in 300 ml. of D/5/W. Titrate by microdrip to lower pressure below 200 and/or diastolic pressure under 120 (usually about 400 ug/minute is needed). Get cyanide levels every 8 hours and discontinue if cyanide is over 10.

<u>or alternatively</u>

1b. Reserpine, 2.5 mg. I.M. every 12 hours. (Diazoxide and nitroprusside have made this a poor third choice because of poor absorption.)

1c. Trimethaphan (Arfonad), 10 mg/minute I.V., to turn by microdrip at rate to keep pressure under 200/140.

2. Start hypertensive management program as directed, using hydralazine, trimethaphan, reserpine, methyldopate, and pentolinium.

NOTES

PULMONARY ARTERY DIASTOLIC PRESSURE LESS THAN 3 -- MORE THAN 18

With the exception of when there is lung disease, the pulmonary diastolic pressure is equivalent to the wedge pressure which, in turn, is equivalent to the left auricular pressure, so, to save the functionability of the balloon-directed catheter, when serial readings are being taken initially -- compare the PA diastolic pressures with the wedge pressures, comparing the waves (page 169), and if the waves jibe with the illustrations (page 171) and the pulmonary diastolic pressure does equal the wedge -- use the pulmonary diastolic pressure and only wedge once or twice a day to be sure they remain the same. This will prolong functionability of your balloon-directed catheter.

ACTIVE CONTINGENCY ORDERS FOR PULMONARY ARTERY DIASTOLIC PRESSURE IF UNDER 5:

Give fluids at rate of 500 to 1000 cc. per hour until pulmonary artery diastolic pressure is over 5.

ACTIVE CONTINGENCY ORDERS FOR PULMONARY ARTERY DIASTOLIC PRESSURE OVER 18 OR FOR RISE OF 5 IN HOUR IF ORIGINAL OVER 10. TO BE DONE UNDER PHYSICIAN'S ORDERS:

1. Digitalize patient (see system on page 196)

2. Give 50 mg. of edecrin I.V.

3. Slow fluids to 50 cc. per hour until pulmonary artery diastolic pressure starts to fall.

4. Give morphine, gr. 1/6 I.M., if blood gases are normal as a pretreatment of the pulmonary edema which should develop shortly.

See page 169 for discussion of flow-directed catheters.

NOTES

PULMONARY ARTERY SYSTOLIC PRESSURE OVER 28

(See page 169 for general information regarding flow-directed catheters.)

Pulmonary artery systolic pressure over 28 means the patient is in heart failure or that because of edema, emboli, fluid overload, or vasoconstriction, there is increased resistance in the pulmonary circulation.

DIAGNOSTIC CONTINGENCY ORDERS FOR PULMONARY ARTERY SYSTOLIC PRESSURE OVER 28:

1. Chest x-ray

2. Cardiac output

3. Wedge pressure

4. Lung scan

5. Blood volume

6. Blood gases

7. EKG

8. Peripheral resistance

ACTIVE CONTINGENCY ORDERS FOR PULMONARY ARTERY SYSTOLIC PRESSURE OVER 28:

Treat for pulmonary emboli if the following data pattern emerges:

1. Chest x-ray   -- abnormal.

2. Cardiac output   -- normal.

3. Wedge pressure   -- under 20.

4. Lung scan   -- abnormal.

5. Blood volume   -- normal.

6. Blood gases   -- abnormal.

7. EKG   -- abnormal with right heart strain pattern.

8. LDH c̄ isoenzymes   -- abnormal.

Do this by following appropriate CONTINGENCY ORDERS for the determinations that are abnormal.

The patient will have had a PULMONARY EMBOLUS under the following circumstances:

1. Abnormal PaO_2.

2. Abnormal lung scan.

3. Rise in LDH isoenzymes.

4. Abnormal chest x-ray.

5. Right access deviation on EKG.

If these criteria are met, use pulmonary embolism system on page 189.

WEDGE PRESSURE ABOVE 18 OR +5 CHANGE IN AN HOUR

(See page 169 for explanation of flow-directed catheters.)

To all intents and purposes a wedge pressure above 18 or a +5 change in an hour means that the left ventricle is not able to pump out all of the blood it is receiving--that is to say the heart is failing. Conversely, a wedge pressure of under 5 means that the patient is hypovolemic.

DIAGNOSTIC CONTINGENCY ORDERS FOR WEDGE PRESSURE ABOVE 18 OR +5 IN AN HOUR:
1. Compare wedge and pulmonary artery diastolic pressures--they should be the same. If that is so, the reading is confirmed.

2. Get cardiac output and peripheral resistance.

3. Chest x-ray.

4. EKG.

5. Hourly urine output.

6. Monitor heart.

ACTIVE CONTINGENCY ORDERS FOR WEDGE PRESSURE ABOVE 18 OR +5 IN AN HOUR:
1. Digitalize the patient (page 196).

2. Give edecrin, 50 mg. I.V.

3. Slow fluids to 50 ml. per hour until wedge pressure starts to fall.

4. Give morphine, gr. 1/6 I.M., if patient does NOT have chronic pulmonary disease.

WEDGE PRESSURE UNDER 5

A low wedge pressure means either that you are not wedging properly or that the patient is hypovolemic.

DIAGNOSTIC CONTINGENCY ORDERS FOR WEDGE PRESSURE UNDER 5:

1. Compare P.A. curve with wedge curve to be sure you are wedging properly.

2. Get blood volume.

3. Check for bleeding:
   a. Rectal (black stool)
   b. Hematocrit
   c. Hemoglobin

4. Check for dissecting aneurysm:
   a. Chest x-ray
   b. Ultrasound for abdomen

ACTIVE CONTINGENCY ORDERS FOR WEDGE PRESSURE UNDER 5:

1. Give fluids at rate of 500 to 1000 ml. per hour until wedge pressure is over 5.

PERIPHERAL RESISTANCE MORE THAN 2000

Peripheral resistance is determined by dividing the mean arterial blood pressure by the cardiac output and including some constants which need not concern us here.

If peripheral resistance is greater than 2000 it is indicative of significant peripheral vasoconstriction that is not letting blood through the smaller vessels. *

DIAGNOSTIC CONTINGENCY ORDERS FOR PERIPHERAL RESISTANCE MORE THAN 2000:

This will be covered by other CONTINGENCY ORDERS.

ACTIVE CONTINGENCY ORDERS FOR PERIPHERAL RESISTANCE MORE THAN 2000:

1. Nipride (sodium nitroprusside), 50 mg. in 500 ml. D/5/W (100 ug/ml), microdripped by piggyback into a running I.V. at rate to decrease systolic blood pressure by 10 mg. mm. (Do NOT run in over 4 ml. per minute.) Titrate the rate of nitroprusside by adjusting the microdrips to a rate that will decrease the systolic blood pressure by 10. If you have a vasopressor such as norepinephrine or dopamine running at the same time, turn this off while you titrate the nipride, and then turn it back on at a rate to get the systolic pressure back up to 90. What you are doing in this case is utilizing the nipride to prevent peripheral vasoconstriction caused by shock and the vasopressor, while still getting maximum benefit from the heart muscle-stimulating effect of the adrenalin-derived compound.

2. Get cyanide levels every 6 hours while patient is on nipride and discontinue it if the level is over ___10___ . **

* Determine peripheral resistance by using nomogram page for peripheral resistance (35).

** 100 if results reported per liter.

NOTES

CARDIAC INDEX ABOVE 4

The cardiac index corrects cardiac output for the size of the patient by dividing the cardiac output in liters per minute by the body surface area of the patient.

Cardiac outputs are easily determined by the thermodilution method, which is done by injecting cold saline into the vena cava and reading the cardiac output by direct readout on an Edwards computer.

If cardiac index is above 3.5 there is a hyperdynamic circulation and the heart is pumping out more blood than usual. This often happens in stressful situations.

DIAGNOSTIC CONTINGENCY ORDERS WHEN CARDIAC INDEX ABOVE 3.5:
1. If the pulmonary artery diastolic pressure is under 18, ignore and treat patient's underlying disease.

2. If there is no obvious reason for the high output, draw serum iodine and thiamine levels. (Hyperthyroidism and beriberi heart disease are two diseases common in high output states).

ACTIVE CONTINGENCY ORDERS WHEN CARDIAC INDEX ABOVE 3.5:
1. If there is no obvious reason for the high output and there is any reason to believe there is dietary deficiency, give thiamine, 500 mg. I.V., every 2 hours x 6. (This will give a dramatic result in beriberi heart disease.)

2. If the serum bound iodine is markedly elevated and there is no other reason apparent for the hyperactive circulation, give reserpine, 2.5 mg. I.M., and oral inderol, 20 mg. by mouth four times a day.

CARDIAC INDEX BELOW 2.5 -- THE HEART, BY DEFINITION, IS IN FAILURE

DIAGNOSTIC CONTINGENCY ORDERS WHEN THE CARDIAC INDEX IS BELOW 2.5:

1. Rule out myocardial infarction by:
    a. EKG

    b. CPK every 6 hours x four, then daily (isoenzymes if abnormal).

    c. SGOT daily x three

2. If no obvious reason for heart failure and patient did not have coronary, rule out pericardial effusion by:
    a. Ultrasound of cardiac area

    b. Heart scan compared to chest x-ray

    c. Comparison of systolic blood pressure on deep inspiration and on deep expiration--more than 20 mm. of mercury difference on expiration means a paradoxical pulse, that is, fluid in the pericardium increases cardiac output when patient takes a deep breath.

3. Rule out fluid overload by blood volume and pulmonary artery diastolic pressure reading.

4. Start Cardiac Flowsheet (page 29).

ACTIVE CONTINGENCY ORDERS FOR CARDIAC INDEX BELOW 2.5:
1. Digitalize by Digitalis System (page 196).

2. Reduce fluid intake to 50 ml. per hour

3. Give edecrin, 50 mg. I.V.

4. Give morphine, gr. 1/6 I.M., if blood gases are normal

5. Be sure the patient is sitting well propped up

6. If patient is in shock and has decreased cardiac output, use the Cardiogenic Shock System (page 179).

DIGOXIN LEVEL UNDER 1.5[*]

This usually means your patient is <u>under</u> digitalized. Follow digitalization schedule of the DIGITALIS SYSTEM: (page 196)

Level	Dose	
2.5	0	Have K 4 or over.
2.0 -- 2.5	0.125	Halve dose if BUN
1.6 -- 1.9	0.25	over 25 or age
1.0 -- 1.5	0.50	over 65.
1.0	0.75	

If--in 2 days--level is not rising, INCREASE the dose schedule one notch, i.e., 1.0 -- 1.5 = 0.75

DIGOXIN LEVEL OVER 2.5

This is usually approaching <u>toxic</u> range.

DIAGNOSTIC CONTINGENCY ORDERS FOR DIGOXIN LEVEL OVER 2.5:
1. Get K

2. Monitor

3. Get calcium

ACTIVE CONTINGENCY ORDERS FOR DIGOXIN LEVEL OVER 2.5:
1. Hold dose of digoxin

2. Increase K to 4.5 if any other signs of toxicity

3. Hold calcium

4. React to arrhythmias as on pages 212-219.

[*] If digoxin levels are not available to you use saliva calcium levels. Levels over 9 should alert you to digitalis intoxication. Arch. Int. Med. 135:1029-1031

SERUM GLUTAMIC PYRUVIC TRANSAMINASE OVER 30

This is the most sensitive parenchymal liver dysfunction.

DIAGNOSTIC CONTINGENCY ORDERS FOR SGPT UNDER 30:

1. Prothrombin time

2. Alkaline phosphatase fractionated

3. Serum bilirubin 1" and total

4. Australian antigen

5. LDH with isoenzymes

ACTIVE CONTINGENCY ORDERS FOR SGPT OVER 30:

1. Institute "hepatitis" precautions if patient is jaundiced.

2. Discontinue hepatotoxic drugs (the tetracyclines, testosterone, and methotrexate are common offenders).

DIAGNOSTIC CONTINGENCY ORDERS FOR SERUM BILIRUBIN OVER 2:

1. SGPT

2. LDH

3. Serum bilirubin 1" and total

4. Alkaline phosphatase

5. Flat plate of abdomen

6. Coombs test

7. LE prep

8. Stool for urobilinogen

ACTIVE CONTINGENCY ORDERS FOR SERUM BILIRUBIN OVER 2:

Treat the cause of the jaundice, which will be revealed by the above tests.

NOTES

HEMATOCRIT LESS THAN 20 OR HEMOGLOBIN LESS THAN 10.5

If the hematocrit is less than 20 or the hemoglobin is less than 10.5, your patient needs red blood cells.

DIAGNOSTIC CONTINGENCY ORDERS FOR HEMATOCRIT LESS THAN 20 OR HEMOGLOBIN LESS THAN 10.5:

1. Check for bleeding by rectal exam, looking for tarry stools.

2. Check list of drugs that can cause anemia (page 192). If the patient is on any of these drugs, get the appropriate test.

3. Check for acquired hemolytic anemia by ordering:
   a. Coombs test--direct and indirect.

   b. Reticulocyte count.

   c. Indirect bilirubin.

4. Check for blood dyscrasia by ordering differential blood cell count.

5. If there is generalized bleeding--use System of Analysis of Bleeding Diathesis outlined on page 204.

6. Check for disseminated intravascular clotting by getting platelet count, prothrombin time, fibrinogen level, fibrin split products, and Lee-White test of clotting time.

7. Get blood culture to rule out endocarditis.

8. For unexplained drop in hematocrit put down nasogastric tube to rule out stress ulcer bleeding.

9. Order serum folate and B_{12} levels.

10. Order a bone marrow examination.

ACTIVE CONTINGENCY ORDERS FOR HEMATOCRIT LESS THAN 20 OR HEMOGLOBIN LESS THAN 10.5:

1. Cell mass if blood volume over 55 ml/kilo until hematocrit is 35 or more

2. Whole blood if blood volume under 55 ml/kilo or if there is obvious active bleeding.

3. If anemia unexplained, STOP drugs listed on page 192 until picture clarifies.

4. If the patient is having intractable bleeding from more than one surface--give two units of fresh frozen plasma, 50 mg. of mephyton I.V., and platelet concentrate (IF platelets under 50,000). Follow System of Analysis of Bleeding Diathesis (page 204).

5. If stab count is over 80, temperature over 102° F., and blood culture positive for Staphylococcus, start Acute Staph Endocarditis program (page 142).

6. If fresh blood comes from nasogastric tube, start Stress Ulcer System (page 161).

7. If prothrombin down, platelets down, fibrinogen down, and fibrin split products up--treat for Disseminated Intravascular Coagulation (page 211).

WHITE BLOOD COUNT (WBC) OVER 15,000

We will assume you will know if your patient has leukemia and if he does NOT, a WBC above 15,000 usually means infection. A rising WBC over 15,000 often means pus is collecting somewhere.

DIAGNOSTIC CONTINGENCY ORDERS FOR WHITE BLOOD COUNT OVER 15,000:

1. Culture blood, urine, sputum, stool, and any wound drainage.

2. If there is stiffness of the neck with no obvious cause, and fever, a lumbar puncture should be done to rule out meningitis.

3. If no overt cause is found and the patient is febrile, order a gallium scan to try to find focus in liver, spleen, mediastinum, or abdomen.

4. If no overt cause is found, have ultrasound of abdomen done to rule out masses or abscesses.

5. If the differential count shows an eosinophile percentage of over 6 per cent, consider drug allergy as cause of the rise.

6. Get G.I. x-rays to rule out empyema of gallbladder and/or colitis.

ACTIVE CONTINGENCY ORDERS FOR WHITE BLOOD COUNT OVER 15,000:

NO ORDERS -- I would never treat solely on the basis of a high WBC. The above diagnostic contingency orders should lead you to a reasonable specific treatment.

WHITE BLOOD COUNT (WBC) BELOW 3500

This can occur because of drug toxicity to the bone marrow, overwhelming infection (particularly when due to gram-negative bacteria), viral infections, tumor invasion of the bone marrow, or autoimmune diseases.

DIAGNOSTIC CONTINGENCY ORDERS FOR WHITE BLOOD COUNT BELOW 3500:
1. Culture sputum, wound, urine, blood, nose, and mouth.

2. LE prep or antinuclear antibody determination.

3. Polymorph alkaline phosphatase (distinguishes myelogenous leukemia cells).

4. Viral diagnostic studies that are available to you.

5. Chest x-ray.

ACTIVE CONTINGENCY ORDERS FOR WHITE BLOOD COUNT BELOW 3500:
1. Discontinue all drugs potentially toxic to the bone marrow (page 195).

2. If WBC is below 500 and the patient's underlying problem is due to immunosuppression, use the Immunosuppressed WBC Prophylactic System: (page 205).
   a. Oxacillin, 0.5 mg. by mouth 3 times a day.

   b. Carbenicillin, 0.5 gm. by mouth 3 times a day until WBC goes over 3000.

   c. Flucytosine, one gm. twice a day.

   d. Cultures of nose, throat, and stool Mondays, Wednesdays, and Fridays.

   e. Discontinue all I.M. injections and draw all blood off the subclavian line or with special arm preparation.

PLATELET COUNT LESS THAN 80,000

The platelets are made by megakaryocytes in the bone marrow and are needed for the clotting process. They decrease first when the bone marrow is being damaged and they can be destroyed at a supernormal rate by acquired antibodies or an enlarged spleen.

DIAGNOSTIC CONTINGENCY ORDERS FOR PLATELET COUNT LESS THAN 80,000:
1. Coombs' test for acquired thrombocytopenia, i.e., antibodies

2. Prothrombin time.

3. Fibrinogen.

4. Fibrin split products.

5. WBC.

6. Spleen scan for spleen size.

7. Clotting time.

ACTIVE CONTINGENCY ORDERS FOR PLATELET COUNT LESS THAN 80,000:
1. Discontinue chloramphenicol and any cancer chemotherapeutic agents until reconsideration by the responsible physician.

2. If there is active bleeding and the platelets are under 20,000--order platelet concentrate twice a day until bleeding stops (in chronic situations and where practicable use HLA matched platelets).

3. If, in addition to the low platelets, there is a positive triad from among the following: lower prothrombin time, lower WBC, increasing fibrin split products, lower fibrinogen, increasing clotting time and recal time -- assume diagnosis of disseminating intravascular coagulation (page 211).

NOTES

RETICULOCYTE COUNT GREATER THAN .8%

This means abnormal extra activity of the bone marrow, either due to recent bleeding or to acute destruction of circulating blood cells due to a toxic drug or autoimmune process.

DIAGNOSTIC CONTINGENCY ORDERS WHEN RETICULOCYTE COUNT GREATER THAN .8%:
1. Stool for blood.

2. Coombs' test.

3. Hemoglobin electrophoresis.

4. 26GP activity of red blood cells.

5. ANA antibody titer.

6. Serum bilirubin 1" and total--and, if negative--

7. Red cell survival time with radioactive chromate.

RETICULOCYTE COUNT LESS THAN .2%

Less than .2% reticulocyte count indicates less than normal production of red blood cells by the bone marrow.

DIAGNOSTIC CONTINGENCY ORDERS WHEN RETICULOCYTE COUNT LESS THAN .2%:
1. Get B_{12}, folic acid levels, and a bone marrow aspiration if low reticulocyte count persists for three days running.

ACTIVE CONTINGENCY ORDERS WHEN RETICULOCYTE COUNT LESS THAN .2%:
1. Discontinue drugs potentially able to depress bone marrow (most likely ones are most anticancer drugs, chloramphenicol, gold salts, sulfa drugs, and butazolidin (page 192).

2. Start daily folic acid, one mg. by mouth, and vitamin B_{12}, 1000 ug. I.M. daily.

NOTES

FIBRINOGEN LESS THAN 250

Fibrinogen is the precursor of fibrin, which is formed in the clotting process. It is formed in the liver and is sometimes elevated in early liver toxemia. However, its main clinical use is the fact that when there is excessive intravascular clotting its level in the blood falls. Therefore it is one of the best indications of intravascular clotting.

DIAGNOSTIC CONTINGENCY ORDERS WHEN FIBRINOGEN IS UNDER 250:

1. Prothrombin time

2. Platelet count

3. WBC

4. Clotting time

ACTIVE CONTINGENCY ORDERS FOR TRIAD OF ABNORMAL CLOTTING TESTS:

If, in addition to the lowered fibrinogen, there is a triad of abnormal values among the four other tests ordered, manage disseminated intravascular coagulation (DIC) as outlined on page 211.

NOTES

PROTHROMBIN TIME MORE THAN 15 SECONDS OR LESS THAN 40%

Prothrombin is a precursor of thrombin, which is used in the clotting process. It is the indicator of the effectiveness of coumadin, and if it is markedly elevated one must always suspect a large dose of coumadin as the cause. However, if this is not the case, its being lowered is another indicator of disseminated intravascular clotting and/or liver failure.

It should always be reported in <u>seconds</u> but many laboratories still use <u>per cent</u> of normal. This is confusing because the numbers are in the same range but go in opposite directions--that is, prothrombin time <u>going from 15 to 25 seconds means prothrombin deficiency</u> while going from 15 to 25 <u>per cent means increasing prothrombin activity.</u> Therefore, ALWAYS know whether reading is in <u>seconds</u> or <u>per cent.</u>

DIAGNOSTIC CONTINGENCY ORDERS FOR PROTHROMBIN TIME OF MORE THAN 15 SECONDS OR LESS THAN 40%:

1. Order SGPT, LDH, and alkaline phosphatase.

2. Order platelets, WBC, clotting time, and fibrin split products.

ACTIVE CONTINGENCY ORDERS FOR PROTHROMBIN TIME OF MORE THAN 15 SECONDS OR LESS THAN 40%:

1. If, in addition to a lowered prothrombin time, there is a positive triad from among the following: lower platelets, lower WBC, increasing fibrin split products, lower fibrinogen, increasing clotting time, and recal time-- assume diagnosis of disseminating intravascular coagulation and manage as outlined on page

2. Check page 193 for drugs that will increase prothrombin time and hold those drugs until physician has been notified.

NOTES

BLOOD UREA NITROGEN (BUN) OVER 20

This means that in all probability the kidneys are functioning at least two-thirds below normal.

DIAGNOSTIC CONTINGENCY ORDERS WHEN BUN IS OVER 20:

1. 24-hour urine for albumin, Na excretion, and K excretion.

2. Creatinine clearance and creatinine level.

3. Serum and urine osmolality.

4. Urinalysis to be looked at for "renal failure" cells and casts.

5. Midstream bacterial count of urine.

6. Infusion I. V. P. with postvoiding x-ray (if BUN under 35 -- above that retro-pyelogram might be necessary to determine cause of problem).

7. Hourly urine output.

8. Blood volume.

9. Urine sodium concentration. A rise in urine sodium is often the first sign of tubular damage to the kidney and should lead to reconsideration of ALL nephrotoxic drugs being given the patient.

10. Check for recent G.I. bleeding since an unexplained BUN rise is often caused by an undiagnosed G.I. bleed. A finger in the rectum can show the tarry stool and solve this problem -- as will putting down a nasogastric tube.

11. If the rise in BUN is sudden, serum K should be checked twice a day and CONTINGENCY ORDERS for K followed.

ACTIVE CONTINGENCY ORDERS FOR BUN OVER 20:

1. Check all medications and adjust all potentially nephrotoxic antibodies (pages 194, 195).

2. Check recent blood transfusions and be sure a recent transfusion reaction did not occur. Have cross matches and typing rechecked.

3. Check hourly urine output and follow CONTINGENCY ORDERS on page 113.

4. If urinary output is above 50 ml. per hour, increase fluid intake to achieve output of up to 200 cc. per hour. The heart rate is the best indicator of pushing fluids too fast unless you have a pulmonary artery catheter in place, in which instance you can push fluids until the pulmonary diastolic pressure rises over 8 ml. of mercury. Increasing the urine output is the best way to "wash down" temporarily elevated BUN.

5. If the BUN is chronically elevated, follow the System for Chronic Failure which includes a low protein diet, fluid excess orally, and amphojel to absorb anions from the G.I. tract.

BLOOD UREA NITROGEN (BUN) UNDER 10

Changes in BUN, even when they occur under the 10 range, are of importance, i.e., if the BUN rises from 8 to 16 this may be the first sign of kidney toxicity due to an antibiotic.

BUN under 8 often means the patient has cirrhosis and is unable to manufacture urea.

DIAGNOSTIC CONTINGENCY ORDERS WHEN BUN IS UNDER 8:
1. Order liver function tests:
   a. SGPT.

   b. Prothrombin time.

   c. Alkaline phosphatase.

   d. Serum bilirubin, one minute and total.

NOTES

CREATININE CLEARANCE LESS THAN 60 OR DECREASE OF 20

This is the most sensitive of kidney function tests and also one of the most accurate--as long as you make sure you correctly time the duration of the urine collection. It indicates the effective blood flow to the kidney and will become abnormal before the BUN rises. An 8-hour, or even 4-hour, creatinine clearance is as accurate as a 24-hour creatinine clearance if the time elapsed between start and finish of urine collection is meticulously recorded.

DIAGNOSTIC CONTINGENCY ORDERS FOR CREATININE CLEARANCE UNDER 60 OR A DECREASE OF 20 FROM A PREVIOUS READING:

1. Institute hourly urine outputs.

2. Get blood levels of gentamicin and of any other antibiotics that are available in your laboratory.

ACTIVE CONTINGENCY ORDERS FOR CREATININE CLEARANCE UNDER 60 OR A DECREASE OF 20 FROM PREVIOUS READING:

1. Discontinue all nephrotoxic drugs until they are specifically reordered by a physician who knows the kidneys may be in trouble.

2. Follow system outlined under BUN OVER 20 (page 113).

NOTE: Creatinine itself is an important laboratory value and increasingly its level, rather than the BUN, is being used to monitor nephrotoxic antibiotics. I personally still use BUN because it is more readily available and it rarely is elevated for extra renal reasons such as a G.I. bleed.

Determine the creatinine-BUN ratio and, if it is over 15:1, the elevated BUN may be extra renal in origin.

One rule of thumb you can use to prevent damage from nephrotoxic antibiotics is to divide the daily dose of the antibiotic by the serum creatinine level.

118

SERUM OSMOLALITY ABOVE 335

This value represents the amount of material in the serum that will cause a change in the freezing point of water and of course these materials build up when the kidneys are not functioning properly or when ineffective anaerobic metabolism in the cells causes a buildup of abnormal metabolites such as lactic acid. When the serum osmolality goes up and the urine osmolality stays low, it means the kidneys are not doing their job of cleaning the blood of inordinate solute. When serum osmolality is over 335 there is too much electrolyte or sugar in the blood. If it is due to D.B.I. the lactic acid elevation and history give the tipoff (page 68).

DIAGNOSTIC CONTINGENCY ORDERS WHEN THE SERUM OSMOLALITY IS ABOVE 335:

1. Check serum sodium.

2. Check blood sugar.

3. Draw lactic acid.

4. Get blood volume.

5. Get urine sodium (under 20 means severe dehydration).

ACTIVE CONTINGENCY ORDERS WHEN THE SERUM OSMOLALITY IS ABOVE 335:

1. Follow orders indicated under Na, blood sugar, and lactic acid (pages 68, 123, 125, 133, 135).

2. Change all fluids to D/5/W and do not try to rehydrate the patient too rapidly because if there is too much intracellular sodium and the cells absorb water, they will swell inordinately and cause brain edema.

NOTES

URINE OSMOLALITY UNDER 250

This usually means the patient is putting out urine that is too dilute, either because the patient's kidneys are not concentrating, or because the patient has just been given a powerful diuretic, or has been overloaded with fluid, or he has early tubular damage. Chronic tubular damage will also cause a low urine osmolality.

DIAGNOSTIC CONTINGENCY ORDERS FOR URINE OSMOLALITY UNDER 250:
1. Blood volume and follow CONTINGENCY ORDERS in its regard (pages 78, 79).

2. Urine concentration test, i.e., get urine osmolality--HOLD fluids for 8 hours--and repeat urine osmolality. If the osmolality does NOT go up over 500 the kidneys are concentrating properly (this can only be done if the patient can stand 8 hours without fluid).

3. Serum sodium and urine sodium.

4. Kidney function panel, i.e., BUN, creatinine clearance, urinalysis, renal failure cells.

5. Hourly urine output.

6. Specifically ask patient about thirst.

ACTIVE CONTINGENCY ORDERS:
1. Follow CONTINGENCY ORDERS regarding inappropriate ADH (page 125). or diabetes insipidus (page 209) as indicated by inordinate urine output or low sodium.

2. Hold nephrotoxic agents until results of kidney function panel have been attended to.

3. Follow blood volume CONTINGENCY ORDERS (pages 78-79).

NOTES

Na (SODIUM) OVER 150

The most common cause of an elevated serum sodium is severe dehydration, usually due to severe diarrhea; fluid loss through a nasogastric tube; or lack of attention to the daily replacement of insensible fluid loss by D/5/W. The blood volume diagnoses this.

The second cause is salt overload with Ringer's lactate or saline, each of which contains 9 gm. of salt per liter. If the Na rises because of a salt overload there is always another problem such as secondary aldosteronism, because otherwise the excess saline is distributed throughout the body in edema fluid.

The daily salt requirement is not over 18 gm. so more than 2 liters of salt-containing solutions are rarely indicated. A normal blood volume indicates salt load is probably the cause. In burns the excess salt may not be manifest until the excess sodium--which migrates to the muscles--begins to be mobilized as the patient has diuresis.

Another cause of elevated sodium level is the hyperosmolality syndrome which may be caused by a combination of renal tubular damage, hyperaldosteronism, and sodium overload. In this syndrome Na gets into the cells in high concentration and the patient goes into coma. (See page 119 also.)

DIAGNOSTIC CONTINGENCY ORDERS FOR Na OVER 150:

1. Blood volume.

2. Urinary sodium concentration.

3. Urinary K concentration.

4. Urine and serum osmolality.

5. BUN and creatinine clearance.

6. Aldosterone level by radioimmunoassay.

ACTIVE CONTINGENCY ORDERS FOR Na OVER 150:

1. If blood volume under 50 ml/kilo--increase fluid intake with D/5/W, 5 liters per day. (Watch pulmonary artery pressure and pulse rate.)

2. If blood volume is normal and urine sodium is over 40 mEq/liter--increase fluid intake with 4 liters of D/5/W and give Lasix, 60 mg. I.V. every 6 hours.

3. If blood volume is normal and the urine sodium is under 40 mEq/liter --
   a. Aldactone, 25 mg. (down clamped stomach if necessary) every 4 hours and

   b. Lasix, 60 mg. I.V., every 6 hours.

4. If serum osmolality above 350--restrict D/5/W to 3000 ml. over output. (If you give too much fluid load and the kidneys are not putting out Na well, the Na will go into the cells, to their detriment.

5. If Na is rising, osmolality is over 350, and urine output is not adequately getting rid of sodium--I think hemodialysis is the best way out of this dilemma.

Finally, hypernatremia may be "essential" (Arch. Int. Med. 134: 889, 1974) due to a tumor in the hypothalamic region--so, if it is unexplained, look for this.

Na (SODIUM) BELOW 130

Low sodium concentration in the serum is usually due to a combination of water overload and sodium depletion which, in turn, is usually due to the habit many have of maintaining patients on I.V.s of D/5/W. Sodium depletion is best demonstrated by ordering a urine sodium, which will be under 15 mEq/liter of urine, and hypervolemia by a blood volume.

Hypervolemia is a second cause of low serum sodium and this is established by a blood volume.

The third cause of low sodium is the secretion of inappropriate antidiuretic hormone (IADH) which happens in head injury, carcinoma of the lung, severe burns, shock, and from antitumor drugs. The criteria for the diagnosis of IADH are:

1. Serum sodium under 130.

2. Urine sodium over 20 mEq/liter.

3. Plasma osmolality under 290.

4. Normal BUN, blood volume, and serum cortisol.

5. Toxic psychosis.

DIAGNOSTIC CONTINGENCY ORDERS FOR Na UNDER 130:

1. Blood volume.

2. Serum osmolality and urine osmolality.

3. BUN.

4. Serum cortisol.

5. Urine sodium.

ACTIVE CONTINGENCY ORDERS FOR Na UNDER 130:

1. Serum Na under 130 and urine Na under 15--change I.V. fluids to saline.

2. Serum Na under 130 and blood volume over 80 ml/kilo--give edecrin, 50 mg., and change fluid administration to saline.

3. Serum Na under 130 and urine Na over 20, plasma osmolality under 290, with normal BUN, serum cortisol, and blood volume--restrict fluid to 1000 ml. of saline per day, i.e., treat for IADH and hold any cancer chemotherapy for a few days while this straightens out.

4. Serum Na under 130 and serum cortisol under 6--follow orders on page 125.

5. If serum Na under 115 for any reason give 5% saline, 500 ml. I.V. in two hours and monitor. Do not do this in a cirrhotic patient who might be running a chronic hyponatremia, or in an elderly patient who may respond simply to fluid restriction and 500 cc. of saline.

K (POTASSIUM) UNDER 3.8

Diuretics are the most common cause of a low potassium and a good share of the patients entering the hospital who have been on diuretics have too little potassium. A low K will potentiate the action of digitalis so the K level MUST be known before digitalis in any form is used (page 196).

A second cause of a low K is lack of replacement in patients on "nothing by mouth".

The third cause of low K is alkalosis, which drives the K into the cell. All sick patients should be kept at a normal K level because this ion is the most important for intracellular metabolism. K must be particularly watched during hyperalimentation, where the high carbohydrate metabolism is very demanding of K participation as well as phosphate participation (page 177).

DIAGNOSTIC CONTINGENCY ORDERS FOR K UNDER 3.8:
1. 24-hour urine excretion of K--measure it in urine, in drainage, and in suction.

2. Get BUN and creatinine clearance.

3. Get aldosterone level.

4. Repeat electrolyte determination in 8 hours.

5. Monitor EKG--note T wave levels.

6. Digoxin level.

ACTIVE CONTINGENCY ORDERS FOR K UNDER 3.8:
1. Follow Potassium Control System--see page 177

NOTES

K (POTASSIUM) ABOVE 5.5

The most common cause of hyperkalemia is renal failure and elevation of the K level is usually the cause of death in this condition. It can also result from massive intravascular hemolysis such as that resulting from mismatched transfusions. Finally it may be due to the fact that the patient is taking potassium supplements in the face of kidney failure.

The more <u>unusual causes</u> of hyperkalemia are as follows:

Deficient Hormonal Effects	Test
1. Generalized adrenal insufficiency.	Cortisone level.
2. Hypofunction--renin, angiotensin, aldosterone system.	Aldosterone level.
3. Excess spirolactone (aldactone).	From history.
4. Excess dietary intake.	
5. Acidosis (pH $\downarrow$)	
6. Malignant hyperpyrexia.	After anesthesia.
7. Hyperkalemic periodic paralysis.	From history.
8. K-retaining drug such as Trianterene.	From history.
9. Lab error -- blood hemolyzed.	

DIAGNOSTIC CONTINGENCY ORDERS FOR K OVER 5.5:

1. Repeat electrolytes immediately to check for laboratory error, and again in 4 hours.

2. EKG -- note T waves.

3. Hourly urine output.

4. BUN, creatinine clearance.

5. Urinary K.

6. Cortisol level.

7. Aldosterone level.

ACTIVE CONTINGENCY ORDERS FOR K OVER 5.5:

1. Stop all K-containing fluids (Ringer's lactate for one).

2. If there are EKG effects noted--give patient 3 ampules of calcium gluconate I.V. in first hour--to modify these.

3. If EKG changes noted--give 2 ampules of NaHCarb (88 mEq Na) to make alkalotic.

4. Give 50 cc. of 50% glucose every 3 hours. Follow each with 15 units of regular insulin (this uses up K in the metabolism of the glucose).

5. Give Kayexalate (polystyrene sulfonate) down stomach tube--15 gm. 4 times a day. Patients cannot tolerate this by mouth. If this is not practicable, put a 30 ml. Foley catheter in the rectum and give 30 gm. of Kayexalate in sorbitol every 4 hours. Leave in for 30 minutes, then deflate the Foley balloon.

6. Under this program, if urine output is adequate, wash out the excess K by giving I.V. fluids at a rate to keep output over 100 (pulmonary diastolic artery pressure under 20 and pulse under 110) while giving lasix, 40 mg. I.V. every 4 hours. Give D/5/W at rate of 250 ml/hour.

7. If K level approaches 6--have a shunt put in and start hemodialysis, OR, if the patient has a temporary type renal shutdown, consider peritoneal dialysis (page 163).

CALCIUM BELOW 7

The common causes of calcium below 8 are:
1. Small bypass and malabsorption.

2. Hypothyroidism.

3. Renal insufficiency.

4. Acute pancreatitis.

5. Calcitonin producing tumors -- tetany and seizures are the main manifestations.

6. Hypoalbuminemia.

DIAGNOSTIC CONTINGENCY ORDERS FOR CALCIUM BELOW 7:
1. Stool for fat.

2. Phophorus concentration.

3. Serum amylase.

4. Serum calcitonin and parathormone levels by radioimmunoassay.

5. BUN, creatinine clearance, and urinalysis.

6. Total protein in serum. (This may be the reason for the low value which may be due to lack of protein to carry calcium.)

ACTIVE CONTINGENCY ORDERS FOR CALCIUM BELOW 7:
1. GIVE 10 ml. calcium gluconate over 5 minutes time, I.V., every 3 hours until tetany stops and calcium level is <u>over</u> 8.

2. For chronic low calcium due to malabsorption or renal disease, give calcium gluconate, 2 gm. (2 tablets) q.i.d.

3. In renal failure and chronic calcemia give 50,000 units of vitamin D each day.

4. In renal failure give amphojel, 30 cc. by mouth, every 6 hours to absorb phosphates.

CALCIUM ABOVE 10

Hypercalcemia is caused by hyperparathyroidism, mobilization of calcium due to cancer chemotherapy, sarcoidosis, toxic doses of vitamin D, multiple myeloma, or other bone metastases. High calcium can cause respiratory arrest and digitalis toxicity so it must be reacted to briskly.

DIAGNOSTIC CONTINGENCY ORDERS FOR CALCIUM ABOVE 10:

1. Check chest x-ray, x-rays of hands and feet, serum globulin, tuberculin test to rule out sarcoid.

2. Compare calcium and phosphorus and if phosphorus is below 4, get level of hyperparathyroid hormone by immunoassay (it should be under 150).

3. Discontinue any vitamin D and get kidney, ureters, and bladder x-ray (KUB) to rule out calcific kidneys.

4. Discontinue cancer chemotherapy until situation is corrected.

5. 24-hour urine excretions of calcium and phosphorus.

6. Bence-Jones protein in urine and bone scan for multiple myeloma.

7. Serum amylase for pancreatitis.

8. BUN, creatinine clearance, urinalysis, urine and serum osmolalities.

9. Monitor with EKG.

10. Digoxin level.

ACTIVE CONTINGENCY ORDERS FOR CALCIUM ABOVE 10:

1. If calcium above 11 start saline I.V. at rate of 100 ml. per hour and run continuously until calcium level is below 12.

2. If calcium above 12 start prednisolone, 20 mg., 4 times a day. Decrease 10 mg. a day and discontinue when calcium is under 10.

3. Inorganic phosphate, one gm., twice a day if phosphorus level is under 6.

4. If calcium stays above 13 on this program give mithramycin, 0.05 mg/kilo per day for 3 days, checking platelets each day. This is to be used for hypercalcemia after bone metastasis and/or chemotherapy.

5. If calcium level above 13 and any cardiac or clinical problems--DIALYZE.

BLOOD SUGAR BELOW 80

The usual cause of hypoglycemia is insulin or, in a Critical Care Unit, a rebound phenomenon after the patient is taken off hyperalimentation.

DIAGNOSTIC CONTINGENCY ORDERS FOR BLOOD SUGAR BELOW 80:

1. Determine if the patient has been taking insulin and if so, what kind.

2. If not on insulin, get insulin level by radioimmunoassay.

3. Draw cortisol level (adrenal insufficiency occasionally causes significant hypoglycemia).

ACTIVE CONTINGENCY ORDERS FOR BLOOD SUGAR BELOW 80:

1. If the patient is on insulin and he is unconscious or tremulous and sweaty, give 50% glucose, 50 cc. I.V.

2. If diabetic, administer regular insulin on the basis of blood sugar levels until a stable diabetic regimen is possible. After several days and the establishment of relationship between blood sugar and urine sugar, check urine sugar 4 times a day and give regular insulin, 20 units each time urine sugar is 4+.

3. If there is persistent low blood sugar, order a serum insulin level to rule out insulinoma.

4. Occasionally, after hyperalimentation the patient's pancreas will be over-active for a while and cause attacks of hypoglycemia. Multiple feedings of fatty foods cure this.

134

NOTES

BLOOD SUGAR OVER 200

Acutely ill patients often have blood sugar concentrations over 200 and, in fact, with hyperalimentation this is the rule rather than the exception and does not have to be reacted to.

BLOOD SUGARS OVER 300 should result in 20 units of regular insulin, given every 2 hours until the level is below 300.

BLOOD SUGARS OVER 400 should result in 25 units of regular insulin every 2 hours until level is below 300.

BLOOD SUGARS OVER 500 should result in 25 units of regular insulin every hour until trend is downward.

If the patient is in acidosis -- follow the more vigorous schedule given on page 209.

NOTES

CORTISOL LEVEL LESS THAN 5

This determination is particularly helpful in patients who have been resuscitated with corticosteroids and then go on to a lung illness. We usually try to get them off the cortisone preparations and, as the illness drags on, the patient often slips into adrenal insufficiency. Monitoring serum cortisol at regular intervals will pick this up and allow for maintenance corticosteroid administration.

DIAGNOSTIC CONTINGENCY ORDERS FOR CORTISOL LEVEL LESS THAN 5:
1. 24-hour urine for 17-ketosteroids and ketogenic steroids.

2. Blood sugar.

3. Give ACTH, 20 mg. I.M. and check level of cortisol one hour later.

ACTIVE CONTINGENCY ORDERS FOR CORTISOL LEVEL LESS THAN 5:
1. Give hydrocortisone, 20 mg. in next I.V.

2. Give prednisolone, 5 mg. by mouth 3 times a day (if the patient is on NPO put this in the I.V.) for the next week, then check for adrenal insufficiency again.

3. Give supplementary carbohydrate as needed to keep blood sugar over 80.

TEMPERATURE OVER 104° OR LESS THAN 96°

The cooling blanket has proven an effective tool to control body temperature and it should be used to keep the temperature under 104°. Similarly, it can be used to bring the temperature up to 96°. Extreme temperature variations of these sorts are always significant and their causes must be sought. In unexplained hypothermia, gram-negative shock is always a prime candidate as the cause. It should be revealed by other tests of the Critical Care package. If the stab count is greater than 75%, therapy for gram-negative shock should be started (page 174).

PERCENT OF STABS (i.e., NONSEGMENTED YOUNG POLYMORPHONUCLEAR
LEUKOCYTES)

Since severe infection can cause either a very high or a very low white blood
count, THE PER CENT OF STABS SEEMS TO BE THE BEST INDICATOR OF SEP-
SIS. A rise of over 20% in the stabs usually means the patient is developing a
severe infection.

DIAGNOSTIC CONTINGENCY ORDERS IF PER CENT OF STABS OVER 65% OR A
RISE IN PERCENTAGE OF OVER 20%:
  1. Culture blood, stool, sputum, urine, and wound drainage unless site of
     infection is obvious.

ACTIVE CONTINGENCY ORDERS IF PER CENT OF STABS OVER 65% OR A RISE
IN PERCENTAGE OF OVER 20%:
  1. If patient has temperature of over 101° F., tachycardia, and is hypoten-
     sive -- start program for gram-negative shock (page 174).

  2. If culture results are back, follow treatment schedule indicated by these
     results (page 142-145).

  3. If patient is immunodepressed and under cancer therapy, treat for Pseudo-
     monas and Staphylococcus infection (page 143 and 142).

NOTES

PATHOGENIC MICROORGANISMS

Detailed discussion of the treatment of infection is outside the scope of this manual but since it is one of the author's favorite subjects a brief discussion will follow.

At present, in Critical Care Units across the world, twelve species of micro-organisms cause the vast majority of the problems, with several other species appearing in patients who are immunodepressed, either as part of their cancer chemotherapy or transplant maintenance program. These organisms all may be considered normal flora and are carried by most people, so a positive culture in itself does not mean the patient has an infection.

The code used to identify these organisms on the Critical Care Flowsheet is as follows:

Source	Symbol
Blood	B
Urine	U
Sputum, tracheal aspirate, or bronchial brush specimen	S
Wound	W

Organisms: "The Big Twelve"	Symbol
1. Coagulase-positive Staphylococcus	S+
2. Proteus	P
3. Pseudomonas aeruginosa	Ps.
4. Klebsiella aerobacter	KA
5. Escherichia coli	EC
6. Fungi	
a. Candida albicans	CA
b. Aspergillosis	AS
c. Histoplasma	HI
d. Blastomyces	BL
e. Coccidioides	CC
7. Bacteroides	BA
8. Serratia marcescens	SM
9. Herpes group (including cytomegalic inclusion disease)	HG
10. Herellia	H
11. Clostridia group	CL
12. Pneumocystis carinii	PC

Thus, in the code on the Critical Care Flowsheet "BS+" means a blood culture positive for coagulase-positive Staphylococci.

SYSTEM FOR
ANTIBIOTIC TREATMENT OF INFECTION BASED ON RESULTS OF CULTURES

ACTIVE CONTINGENCY ORDERS FOR POSITIVE CULTURES OF THE 12 MOST COMMON AND VIRULENT MICROORGANISMS SEEN IN A CRITICAL CARE UNIT:

In each case, before these orders are instituted an M.D. decision that an infection does indeed exist must be made. It will be based on the appearance of the patient, the stab count, pulse, temperature, blood pressure, and physical examination. The automatic "Fail-Safe" for each antibiotic mentioned is detailed in the remarks concerning them in the drug briefs (page 191). How long treatment should be continued or whether it should be changed will depend in each case on clinical response and sensitivity tests. This section will be controversial and is based on the author's experience and research activities of the past 25 years.

1. Coagulase-positive Staphylococcus: This organism is present in 70% of the people in the world so a positive culture per se with no evidence of infection does not indicate the need for treatment.

   Moderate infection: All Staphylococci are sensitive to oxacillin and a moderate infection will respond to:
   a. Oxacillin, 0.5 mg. by mouth, 4 times a day
   b. If the patient is penicillin-hypersensitive, lincomycin, 0.5 gm. by mouth 4 times day, is the second choice.

   Overwhelming infection such as acute bacterial endocarditus: It seems reasonable to attack overwhelming Staphylococci at more than one metabolic site. Accordingly, for an overwhelming Staphylococcal endocarditis or pneumonia or peritonitis or meningitis, give in the first 24 hours:
   a. Methicillin, 12 gm. in 500 ml. of D/5/W
   b. Lincomycin, 6 gm. in 500 ml. of D/5/W
   c. Gentamicin, 100 mg. in 500 ml. of D/5/W
   d. Gamma globulin*, 20 cc. in 500 ml. of D/5/W   (cont'd)

---

* Waisbren, B.A.: Pyogenic Osteomyelitis and Arthritis of the Spine Treated with Combinations of Antibiotics and Gamma Globulin. J. Bone & Joint Surg. 42:414, 1960.

2. Proteus: This organism will cause chronic urinary tract infections and should be eradicated if possible from the urine because of its propensity to cause stone formation. One subspecies of Proteus, P. morgani, is sensitive to the penicillins and penicillin and chloramphenicol potentiate each other against Proteus organisms.

Moderate Proteus infections:
a. Ampicillin, 0.5 gm. by mouth, 4 times a day
b. Chloramphenicol, 0.5 gm. by mouth, 4 times a day

Overwhelming Proteus infections: Gram-negative shock, ruptured viscus, meningitis, pneumonia:
a. Chloramphenicol, 8 gm., and gamma globulin, 10 cc., in 500 ml. of saline
b. Penicillin, 10 millions units, I.V., in 500 ml. of D/5/W
c. Gentamicin*, 150 mg., I.V. in 500 ml. of D/5/W

3. Pseudomonas aeruginosa: This is an unusually benign organism except when the patient is burned, has leukemia, or is under immunodepression. In these cases it becomes virulent and often kills the patient.

Moderate Pseudomonas infection:
a. Carbenicillin, 0.35 gm. by mouth, 4 times a day. No other oral medications will be effective in treating a Pseudomonas infection.

Severe Pseudomonas infection (burn, pneumonia, endocarditis, meningitis):
a. Polymyxin B, 150 mg., and gamma globulin, 10 cc., I.V. in one liter of saline
b. Carbenicillin, 10 gm., I.V. in one liter of saline
c. Tobramycin, 150 mg., I.V. in 500 ml. of saline

(cont'd)

* The other aminoglycoside antibiotics such as tobramycin and kanamycin may be used here in correct dosage, but in my opinion they probably are more toxic than gentamicin.

4. Klebsiella-Aerobacter group: This group of gram-negative bacilli have the highest variability regarding their sensitivities to antibiotics and it is in this group that sensitivity tests have their greatest value.

Moderate Klebsiella infections: In the urinary tract use either:
a. Ampicillin, 0.5 mg. by mouth, 4 times a day -- OR
b. Macrodantin, 50 mg. by mouth, 4 times a day

Change if sensitivity tests indicate it.

In other sites and outside the hospital use:
c. Oxytetracycline (terramycin), 0.5 gm. by mouth, 3 times a day, is usually effective

Overwhelming Klebsiella infections:
a. Chloramphenicol*, 8 gm., and gamma globulin, 10 cc., I.V. in 500 ml. of saline
b. Gentamicin, 150 mg., I.V. in 500 ml. of saline

5. Escherichia coli: This organism is usually sensitive to most antibiotics.

Moderate Escherichia coli infections: In the urinary tract use either:
a. Bactrium, 0.5 gm. by mouth, 4 times a day -- OR
b. Macrodantin, 50 mg. by mouth, 4 times a day

Other than urinary or outside the hospital use:
c. Oxytetracycline (terramycin), 500 mg. by mouth, 4 times a day

Severe Escherichia coli infections:
a. Chloramphenicol, 8 gm. I.V. in 500 ml. of saline
b. Gentamicin, 150 mg. I.V. in 500 ml. of saline

(cont'd)

* If you, or your Service, are inordinately afraid of chloramphenicol, substitute keflin or ampicillin, 8 gm., but remember -- chloramphenicol does not cause aplastic anemia anymore frequently than penicillin causes anaphylaxis.

6. Fungi:

   Candida Albicans: This fungus is rarely a pathogen except in immuno-depressed patients but if Candida keep growing out, particularly in the mycelian phase, it may be the cause of the infection.

   A systemic infection with Candida will usually respond well to 15 mg. of amphotericin B daily. Start with 5 mg. the first day, 10 mg. the next day, and then continue with 15 mg. per day for 14 days, using the "Fail Safe"'s on page 191.   Use with this flucytosine, 500 mg. by mouth 4 times a day (page 205).

   Local Candida infections of the mouth respond well to the following: 50 mg. of amphotericin B, dissolved in 200 cc. of "nice" tasting vehicle (your pharmacist will have one). Dab with Q tips all involved areas 4 x a day.

   Severe fungal infections due to Aspergillosis, Histoplasma, Blasto-myces, or Coccidioides should be treated with 35 to 40 mg. of ampho-tericin B per day until a total dose of 1.5 to 2 gm. are given. This is to be administered as outlined on page 147.   Flucytosine, 2 gm. per day, is given concurrently.

   Summary of treatment for fungus diseases (see page 147)

7. Bacteroides -- This slender anaerobic gram-negative rod is hard to grow but it is the most common pathogen in gastrointestinal catastrophes and postoperative problems. Chloramphenicol is the drug of choice and the empirical observation that this drug gives the best result in intra-abdominal sepsis has kept surgeons using it in spite of dire warnings and threats by nonmedical meddlers. Lincomycin is equally as good but of course does not get the Escherichia coli which are also usually present. Therefore, for severe intra-abdominal sepsis, which usually is due to Bacteroides and E. coli, the following program will be indicated.
   a. Chloramphenicol, 8 gm. I.V. daily in 500 ml. of D/5/W
   b. Lincomycin, 6 gm. I.V. daily in 500 ml. of D/5/W
   c. Gentamicin, 80 mg. I.M. twice the first day and then the dose adjusted by serum level and creatinine level
       (This potentiates both the chloramphenicol and the lincomycin.)

This program should be used for any severe Bacteroides infection be it in the lung, abdominal cavity, or brain.

If there is NOT good response -- hyperbaric oxygen should be added.

NOTES

SUMMARY OF TREATMENT FOR FUNGUS DISEASES

Possible Disease	Diagnostic Test	Therapy
FUNGI -		
1. Candida Albicans	Culture and look - (Myocelial phase associated with virulence)	Amphotericin B* and Flucytosine
2. Blastomycosis	Culture--but better still-- biopsy Complement fixation	" " "
3. Histoplasmosis	Culture--but better still-- biopsy Complement fixation	" " "
4. Coccidioidomycosis	Culture Complement fixation	" " "
5. Phycomycetes (mucormycoses)	Culture Biopsy	" " "
6. Actinomycosis	Anaerobic culture smear	Penicillin--30 million units/day for 6 weeks
7. Nocardia	Aerobic and acid fast on smear	Sulfadiazine

*ORDERS FOR SAFE ADMINISTRATION OF AMPHOTERICIN B

(1) Record BUN, K, hgb, daily input--output, and cumulative dose.

(2) Day 1 -- 1 mg. amphotericin B in 500 ml. of D/5/W with 30 mEq KC1.
Day 2 -- 2 mg. " " " " " " " " " " "
Day 3 -- 5 mg. " " " " " " " " " " "
Day 4 - 10 mg. " " " " " " " " " " "
Day 5 - 15 mg. " " " " " " " " " " "
Day 6 - 20 mg. " " " " " " " " " " "
Day 7 - 25 mg. " " " " " " " " " " "
Day 8 - 30 mg. " " " " " " " " " " "
Day 9 - 35 mg. " " " " " " " " " " "

Continue until 1.5 to 2 gm. total dose.

(3) Follow amphotericin B with $12\frac{1}{2}$ gm. mannitol in 500 ml. D/5/W.
-- Half dose any day BUN up 5 -- cell mass if hemoglobin under 10.

(4) Give 2 gm. flucytosine each day unless platelets go under 100,000.

8. <u>Serratia marcescens</u>: This is almost always caught in the hospital and on <u>minor wounds is not</u> very dangerous and often may be treated with a dab solution.

On the other hand, in immunodepressed or overwhelmingly ill patients it will cause a fatal bacteremia.

Usually it is only sensitive to the aminoglycoside group of antibiotics or the tetracyclines. Sensitivity tests may provide pleasant surprises, such as chloramphenicol sensitivity, so they should always be done.

<u>Mild local infection with Serratia marcescens</u>:
a. Dab solution: one liter of tap water
         1000 mg. of chloramphenicol
         0.5 gm. neomycin
         40 mg. polymyxin B
         40 mg. amphotericin B

<u>Severe infection with Serratia marcescens</u>:
a. Oxytetracycline, 2 gm. I.V. in 500 ml. saline, through subclavian line (check SGPT daily -- see Drug Notes, page 183.)
b. Gentamicin, 80 mg. I.V. in 500 ml. D/5/W 3 times a day initially-- then dose adjusted to level of between 4--6 ug/ml. of serum
c. If on respirator--gentamicin, 4 mg. in 3 ml. bronchosol every 6 hours

9. <u>Herpes group</u>: <u>Cytomegalic inclusion body virus</u>
        <u>Herpes type A</u>
        <u>Herpes type B</u>

A patient in shock and unconscious, with a temporal lobe localization, must be considered to have an acute Herpes encephalitis, which has a terrible prognosis. I treat these with cytosine arabinoside, 100 mg. I.V. STAT and 50 mg. I.V. twice a day for 3 days in conjunction with gamma globulin, 30 cc. This is based on our own <u>in vitro</u> studies. Others use idoxyuridine, 80 mg./day, for this condition but no worker has yet proven effective therapy for Herpes infection. However, I cannot resist sharing my experience with you regarding the occasional successful use of large doses of corticosteroids and/or cytosine arabinoside in cases of overwhelming virus disease.

10. <u>Herellia:</u> These organisms are also usually hospital caught and respond best to:
    a. Gentamicin, 80 mg. I.V. in 500 ml. D/5/W 3 times a day initially, then maintained by daily levels and/or dividing the daily dose of 1.5 mg/kilo by the creatinine level.

    If there is a pulmonary infection, use the gentamicin by aerosol as well.

11. <u>Clostridia group:</u> These fat gram and anaerobic bacilli of course cause <u>gas gangrene.</u> They are all sensitive to penicillin and chloramphenicol, which is why when there is dead tissue inaccessible to air, one of these two drugs should be given prophylactically.

    When a person develops gas gangrene immediate transfer for hyperbaric treatment should be the first thought, since this might make the necessity for surgical debridement minimal (page 243). If this is not available or practicable, the widest excision is necessary to be followed with:
    a. Penicillin G, 20 million units I.V.
    b. Gas gangrene antitoxin, 40,000 units I.V. (of doubtful value, but give it)
    c. Laying in of catheters through which hydrogen peroxide solution is given every 4 hours

    NOTE: These patients, while looking well, go into circulatory collapse, so digitalize them and be prepared for the worst

12. <u>Pneumocystis carinii:</u> This protozoal infection follows immunosuppression <u>and organ transplant.</u> It is hard to demonstrate because these are usually the patients on whom you do not want to do a lung biopsy. Therefore, if bronchial brush is negative and you have a lesion in a patient of this type, you may want to empirically treat it with:
    a. Pentamidine isethionate*, 40 mg. I.M. 3 times a day
    b. Flagyl, 29 mg. by mouth 3 times a day
    c. Pyrimethamine, 25 mg. a day
    d. Trimethoprim/sulfamethoxazole, 2 tablets 3 times a day
    e. Sulfadiazine, 4 gm. per day

These patients will need maximum control, which is why all possibly helpful drugs are suggested--to be given at once. Toxoplasmosis is a less serious disease, caused by a Protozoa-like organism, and will respond to sulfadiazine and daraprim (pyrimethamine) 25 mg./day, monitored by platelet counts.

* Pentamidine is available upon request: Parasitic Drug Service, National Center for Disease Control in Atlanta, Georgia.

NOTES

CONTINGENCY ORDERS SYSTEM FOR CHEST X-RAY FINDINGS

(IF X-RAY FINDINGS ARE POSITIVE, FIND DIAGNOSIS AND REACT ACCORDINGLY)

INCREASE IN HEART SIZE

DIAGNOSTIC CONTINGENCY ORDERS FOR INCREASED HEART SIZE:
Unless all other signs point to development of heart failure:
1. Get EKG.

2. Ultrasound or scan to rule out pericardial effusion.

3. Record systolic blood pressures on inspiration and expiration. If there is over a 20 ml/Hg rise on deep expiration you may have cardiac tamponade ("paradoxical pulse").

4. Get blood gases.

ACTIVE CONTINGENCY ORDERS FOR INCREASED HEART SIZE:
1. If heart failure--digitalize (page 196).

2. If pericardial effusion suspected, get specific order from responsible physician.

3. Slow fluids unless pulmonary artery pressures indicate otherwise (page

DEVELOPMENT OF FLUID IN PLEURAL CAVITY

DIAGNOSTIC CONTINGENCY ORDERS FOR FLUID IN PLEURAL CAVITY:
1. Check CVP or pulmonary artery pressure for heart failure.

2. Get CBC--high WBC will help indicate empyema.

ACTIVE CONTINGENCY ORDERS FOR FLUID IN PLEURAL CAVITY:
1. Digitalize if indicated by pulmonary artery pressure.

2. If WBC is elevated have chest tap done to rule out empyema. Be sure culture, smear, protein determination, and differential cell count are done on the fluid that is removed. Have a tube, with citrate, ready so the fluid will not clot before a differential count can be done; be ready with a fixative in case a pleural biopsy is done at the time of fluid removal. If there is empyema, insert 500 mg. of neomycin in 50 ml. of saline into the chest cavity after the fluid is removed.

HIGH DIAPHRAGM

In this case look for collapsed lung (see below) or something below the diaphragm.

DIAGNOSTIC CONTINGENCY ORDERS FOR HIGH DIAPHRAGM:
1. Flat plate of abdomen.

2. Simultaneous scan of liver and lungs to demonstrate suprahepatic subphrenic abscess.

3. Ultrasound of abdomen.

ACTIVE CONTINGENCY ORDERS FOR HIGH DIAPHRAGM:
1. Put patient with feet lower than head (reverse Trendelenburg).

2. If ileus--put down a nasogastric tube.

3. If subphrenic--arrange for drainage.

PULMONARY INFILTRATION

A new pulmonary infiltration in a patient in a Critical Care Unit is usually either a Staphylococcal or esoteric pneumonia, a pulmonary embolus, or aspiration. If the patient has been transplanted or is immunodepressed, cytomegalic inclusion body pneumonia or Pneumocystis carinii pneumonia must also be considered (page 149).

DIAGNOSTIC CONTINGENCY ORDERS FOR PULMONARY INFILTRATION:
1. Get CBC, sputum culture, tracheal aspirate (if not immunodepressed and no sputum), and blood culture to rule out pneumonia.

2. Get EKG, LDH with enzymes, blood gases, and lung scan to rule out pulmonary embolus.

3. If patient is immunodepressed, get bronchial brush for pneumocystis and cytomegalic virus studies, culture urine for cytomegalic virus, and look at urine sediment for inclusion cells (CMV) (page 148).

ACTIVE CONTINGENCY ORDERS FOR PULMONARY INFILTRATION:
1. If acutely ill with WBC or stab count up, start treatment for an acute Staphylococcal pneumonia with methicillin, 10 gm. I.V. in 500 ml. of D/5/W, and gentamicin, 100 mg. I.V. in 500 ml. of D/5/W.

2. If acutely ill, immunodepressed, and/or if sputum smear shows gram-negative rods, add treatment for Pseudomonas or Klebsiella pneumonia, i.e., polymyxin B, 150 mg. and gamma globulin, 10 cc., in 500 ml. of D/5/W, and chloramphincol, 8 gm. in 500 ml. of D/5/W.

3. If Pneumocystic carinii is demonstrated in an immunodepressed patient, use pentamidine, 40 mg. I.M. every 4 hours and flagyl, 2 mg. by mouth 3 times a day.

4. If cytomegalic inclusion body virus is demonstrated in an immunodepressed patient, start transfer factor and cytosine arabinoside, 100 mg. I.V. daily.

5. If EKG, gases, pulmonary artery pressure, or LDH isoenzymes suggest pulmonary embolus--start heparin, 5000 units I.V. every 6 hours.

COLLAPSED LUNG (PNEUMOTHORAX)

This often happens after a subclavian stick, so always get a chest x-ray after this procedure is done.

DIAGNOSTIC CONTINGENCY ORDERS FOR COLLAPSED LUNG:
1. Blood gases

ACTIVE CONTINGENCY ORDERS FOR COLLAPSED LUNG:
1. Discontinue all positive pressure ventilation (IPPB).

2. Notify physician in charge.

3. If the patient is in acute distress he may have a tension pneumothorax, which you can relieve--until help arrives--by putting a #14 needle into the chest cavity (critical care nurses should get training in doing this occasionally helpful procedure). Better still, a valved #14 needle might be kept on the ward for just this exigency. It will let air out on expiration but not allow air to be sucked in.

NOTES

GUIDELINES FOR ASSISTED VENTILATION

Mechanical assistance of respiration is one of the most life saving aspects of a Critical Care Unit. The choice of a respirator and its exact indications are as amenable to a systematic approach as any other facet of critical care medicine, but the tremendous differences of opinion that surround respirator use indicates that the best system of managing respiratory failure has not surfaced or, if it has, this has not been proven.

Therefore we will give suggested guidelines and leave blank spaces for each Unit to meet the feelings of its responsible physician. We suggest that the respirator should be initially started with a soft endotracheal tube, which can often be left in place undisturbed for the week or ten days that mechanical assistance is necessary. If a tracheostomy is decided upon it can then be done in an Operating Room at a regularly scheduled time. There should be someone trained in putting in an endotracheal tube in all Critical Care Units at all times, and this person should have immediate access to an M.D. anesthesiologist backup. (In my opinion, the anesthesiologists become the most capable of inserting endotracheal tubes.)

Usual indications for mechanical respiration:
1. PAO_2 of under 60 on $F1O_2$ of 100% means the patient will probably die without mechanical respiration. There are reservations and exceptions, of course; these are:
   a. Providing patient is fully digitalized and maximum measures have been taken to treat heart failure and/or pulmonary edema (including measures such as continuous positive airway pressure -- CPAP and PEEP).
   b. Providing patient is not suffering from chronic lung disease and therefore has adapted to the ominous blood gas finding.

2. $PaCO_2$ of over 50 with these reservations and exceptions:
   a. Patient is chronically carrying a high $PaCO_2$.
   b. Only after full measures to increase ventilation have been taken, such as Narcan (if on narcotics), IPPB, exhortation, chest physiotherapy, and discontinuance of all sedation.

Page on which individual Units can put in their indications if they do not accept those on preceding page:

Indications for mechanical respiration on _____
Critical Care Unit are as follows:

1:

2:

3:

ASSISTED VENTILATION WITH A VOLUME RESPIRATOR

Once the decision has been made to start assisted ventilation with a volume respirator the following suggestions regarding setting on the respirator may be of aid:

RATE: Start with IMV (Intermittent Mandatory Ventilation) if possible at a rate of 12 to 14 per minute. With the patient initiating additional breaths you may be able to reduce the amount of sedation necessary to get a nice adaptation.

TIDAL VOLUME: Start with 10 cc. per kilo (154 lb. man will take 700 ml.). A chronic emphysema patient may need considerably more than this.

INSPIRATION: .6 sec. to 1.2 sec.

EXPIRATION: 2 sec. to 4 sec.

CONCENTRATION OF O_2: Contingency order should read "Adjust FIO_2 to lowest concentration that will yield a certain level of PaO_2 -- usually between 70 -- 100". Check this first at hourly intervals and then 2-hourly and etc. The nearer the concentration of FIO_2 that will give a satisfactory PaO_2 to room air the better.

TRACHEAL SUCTIONING: This should be done as often as necessary to keep the airway "sounding dry" and yielding an adequate total volume. Remember, a sudden increase of tracheal secretions often means pulmonary edema and the necessity to slow fluids and give lasix.

PULMONARY END EXPIRATORY POSITIVE (PEEP) and CONTINUOUS POSITIVE AIRWAY PRESSURE (CPAP): have revolutionized the use of volume respirators by making it possible to get O_2 into the blood stream without the need of toxic levels of FIO_2. It seems now that CPAP is rapidly relegating PEEP to historical interest and in the past few months our trend, as with others, seems to be early and larger CPAP with many times obviation of the need of a volume respirator.

PROBLEMS WITH A LOW $PaCO_2$: While other parameters are being maneuvered to get an adequate PaO_2, too low a $PaCO_2$ is often best countered by lengthening of the tubing to create more dead space. This can also be accomplished by a circuit that allows rebreathing or the addition of CO_2.

TOO RAPID LOWERING OF $PaCO_2$: This causes dangerous potassium shifts so, while artificial ventilation is being instituted, K and pH should be checked every 4 hours. K should be kept between 4 and 5 mEq. in the serum, with the following Contingency Orders:

(cont'd)

K Convention for First 16 Hours on Respirator

4-hour level	K by volutrol in 300 ml. in 4 hours (through CVP catheter)
3.0 -- 3.5	100
3.6 -- 4.0	75
4.0 -- 4.5	50
4.5 -- 5.0	20
>5	0

The shift of potassium will be closely tied to the shifts in pH, which in turn should be controlled by the pH (page 71) and HCO_3 (page 66-67) contingencies. Both K and pH problems can usually be avoided if, when a patient with a markedly elevated $PaCO_2$ is put on a respirator, settings are such as to gradually bring down the $PaCO_2$.

Suggestions for adjustments of the following by physicians of the (fill in name of your client)   Critical Care Unit. (Again, if the suggestions on pages 157-58 seem to need amplification, I challenge the physicians concerned to put in writing the system they wish to use on their own unit.)

RATE:

TIDAL VOLUME:

INSPIRATION:

EXPIRATION:

CONCENTRATION OF $F10_2$:

CONTROL OF $PaCO_2$:

CONTROL OF K:

CONTROL OF pH:

NOTES

STRESS ULCER SYSTEM

PREVENTION SYSTEM:

1. If ileus--put down nasogastric tube.

2. Check every hour for bleeding in secretions.

3. Clamp tube one of 4 hours and put down --
   a. Milk, 6 ounces, during first half-hour.
   b. Maalox, 4 ounces, during second half-hour.

4. ALL patients who are eating and are on corticosteroids of any type --
   a. Donnatol before meals and at 9:00 P.M.
   b. Alternate food and milk in small amounts hourly, with 2 ounces of amphojel (if bowels loose) and maalox, 2 ounces (if constipated).
   c. Stool for blood every other day.

5. ALL patients in shock or with nasogastric tubes --
   a. Vitamin A, 50,000 units I.M. daily (protects micin-secreting cells of the stomach).

ACTIVE TREATMENT SYSTEM:

1. Keep hemoglobin over 11 gm. with transfusions if actively bleeding--with cell mass if problem of overload may exist.

2. Keep platelets normal.

3. Get bleeding diathesis panel (page 204) and correct this.

4. Keep nasogastric tube in but clamp 15 minutes of each hour, at which time you can put down ice water and/or thrombin solution (60 ml.).

5. Do NOT stop the corticosteroids if they are vital for other aspects of management. If they can be stopped without damage, do so.

6. If the ice water and thrombin solution do not help, slow drip levophed (4 mg. in one liter of saline, for an hour) which acts as a gastric mucosa styptic pencil.

7. Start vasopressin, 5 units in 500 ml. of saline by microdrip.

8. Start premarin, 30 mg. I.V.

9. If this does not slow bleeding, have a gastroscopy done to see if you have a "pumper" (which means surgery, particularly for an older person.)

10. If gastroscopy is not feasible or not definitive, do mesenteric angiography to identify bleeding vessels in the stomach. If your angiography man can identify them, then he can use vasopressin or thrombin clots by putting them directly into the vessel.

If 9 and 10 are not feasible, surgery should be done at the time that blood replacement, fresh frozen plasma, intragastric tube thrombin, ice water, norepinephrine, vasopressin, and platelets have not been able to stabilize hemoglobin level. Always operate sooner rather than later. (Although I must admit I have not seen a stress ulcer uncontrolled by Nos. 1 through 10 in the last five years.)

HEMODIALYSIS SYSTEM

The actual mechanics of the use of hemodialysis and peritoneal dialysis are clearly outlined in excellent procedure manuals for the hemodialysis machines and on the prepackage set up for peritoneal dialysis. For some reason both of these modalities are underused and each Unit can overcome its initial reluctance to put hemodialysis in its armamentarium by acknowledging the fact that patients themselves can be taught to dialyze themselves at home. As we have discussed elsewhere, we feel every general hospital should have a Chronic Dialysis Program and the director of this program is the logical person to call on to administrate hemodialysis in a Critical Care Unit. Nurses capable of functioning in a Critical Care Unit can easily learn how to dialyze patients and, if the Chronic Dialysis Unit cannot manage to supply personnel, they should be asked to train the critical care nurses in this procedure. (Remember, patients can be trained so there is no reason why nurses cannot be trained.)

Peritoneal dialysis is rarely indicated in my opinion, except for the few cases of acute poisoning where it will help get rid of excess toxic material--in some cases better than will hemodialysis.

In crucially ill patients, shunts for dialysis should be placed at the time of tracheostomy and placement of balloon pump so that dialysis can be started as soon as it is needed.

Acute dialysis should be started when the kidneys fail to the point that the body cannot get rid of potassium, and should be used to help the kidneys get rid of drug overdoses and other poisons. Particular indications are as follows:

1. Acute kidney failure due to shock, nephrotoxic drugs, or autoimmune disease.
2. Control of excess sodium concentrations.
3. Control of life-threatening hypervolemia and hypovolemia.
4. Control of life-threatening calcium imbalance.

There are four variables that can be controlled during the actual dialysis procedure and specific orders regarding their manipulation should be given by the responsible physician during each dialysis. The election of dialysis fluid is rarely a problem. The standard fluid is used for 90% of dialysis. Potassium-free fluid can be used when K level is dangerously high; the low sodium and low potassium fluid can be used for dangerous hypernatremia or hyperosmolality; and the high calcium fluid can be used for hypocalcemia. In cases of very low serum potassium, up to 4 mEq per liter of K can be added to the standard solution.

The dials to be turned vary on each machine but the Instruction Manual, plus a few hour's instruction, make it well within the province of a critical care nurse to handle dialysis. In addition, a few day's assignment to a Chronic Dialysis Unit each six months should be a part of the in-service training of each critical care nurse.

The four variables to be manipulated during dialysis are:

1. Control of the blood flow -- The usual flow rate is 200 ml. per minute but this can be raised to 400 ml. per minute, or even above if it becomes necessary for maintenance of blood pressure. Rather than go to too high a blood flow, it usually is better to add blood or plasmonate to the system.

2. Pressure on outflow line -- Increased pressure on the outflow line will remove fluid from the system. This can be increased from 20 to 200 and a dial should be available on your machine which will calculate how much fluid will be removed per hour. This simple maneuver is the best way I know of to treat the hypervolemia that so often occurs in acute renal failure.

3. Bath temperature -- This is usually kept at 37°C. but can be raised if the patient is chilly and can be lowered a degree or two if the patient is too febrile. The range is 36 to 38 degrees.

4. Dialysate flow rate -- One can change the dialysate fluid more rapidly to shorten the time for an effective dialysis. In cases when poor shunts or a poor cardiac function give a low blood flow rate, one can partially compensate for this by increasing dialysis flow rate to the maximum. The usual dialysate rate is 300. It can be raised to 400 or 500 in cases when the dialysis must be shortened.

DRUGS THAT CAN BE DIALYZED OUT WITH USUAL SOLUTIONS

amphotericin B

barbiturates

bromides

ethylene glycol

glutethimide

methanal

salicylates

thiocyanates

DRUGS THAT CAN BE DIALYZED OUT WITH LIPID DIALYSIS

secobarbitol

phenothiazines

glutethimide

camphor

Call Round the Clock -- The Poison Index System of Fr. Rumack -- 303-893-7771 for information on poisoning and on whether or not a poison is amenable to hemo-dialysis or peritoneal dialysis.

For more details, refer to:

Bennett, W.M., Dinger, I., and Coggins, C.H.: Guide to Drug Usage in Adult Patients With Impaired Renal Function. A Supplement. J.A.M.A. 223: 991-998, February 1973.

NOTES

PARTIAL LIST OF STOCK SOLUTIONS AVAILABLE FOR DIALYSIS (TRAVENOL)

Description	Na	K	Ca	Mg	Cl	Acetate	Dextrose
Standard	134	2.6	2.5	1.5	104.0	36.6	2.5
Potassium Free	134	0	2.5	1.5	101.4	36.6	2.5
Modified Sodium/ Potassium	130	2.0	2.5	1.5	99.0	37.0	2.5
Low Calcium	134	2.6	1.0	1.5	102.5	36.6	2.5
Calcium 3	130	1.0	3.0	1.0	96.0	39.0	2.0
Low Potassium & Low Calcium	134	1.0	1.0	0.5	100.0	36.5	2.5
Potassium & Dextrose	134		2.5	1.5	101.0	37.0	
Soybean Oil dialysis solution							

NOTES

SYSTEM FOR
"SWAN-GANZING" OR THE PRACTICAL USE OF THE PULMONARY ARTERY BALLOON FLOTATION CATHETER

There are so many articles now appearing about the use of this essential modality that this Section will just give practical tips based on experience in using the pulmonary artery catheter on crucially ill patients (burns, gram-negative shock, cardiogenic shock) rather than in a "cath" lab. How the catheter is placed will depend on the previous experience of the physician who places it. My suggestion for the acutely ill patient is that it be placed through a subclavian approach, with the use of a vein dilator placed around the original penetrating needle. Secondly, use the larger size (#7) because the #5 just does not give as good curves or pressures. If the patient has a truly serious disease, put in the thermodilution catheter immediately because you will find the cardiac output determination to be of vital aid in patient management (pages 30, 31, 87, 89). Remember, when you are using a pulmonary artery catheter in a sick patient, the absolute values and the configuration of the curves are not nearly as important as the trends. So, do not get hung up on beautiful curves and pressure readings but get a baseline and see what happens from there on. If you have used these catheters you know beautiful, classic curves are the exception rather than the rule and much time can be wasted with undue manipulation of the catheters when they are giving you the three trends you really want to know--the pulmonary artery diastolic pressure, the pulmonary artery mean pressure, and a wedge pressure.

With this as a background, let us follow our catheter in:

1. ALWAYS test the balloon before you start -- .8 cc for a 5F - 1.5 cc. for a 7F. (There is nothing more frustrating than a catheter in the auricle with a broken balloon).

2. Between 30 to 40 cm. from the anticubital area the catheter tip is in the right atrium and at that point a pressure reading should be 5 cm. of mercury. However, if the patient is hypovolemic, this pressure may be 0 so you will have to tell that you are in the right atrium by the curve--which should be broad. With the balloon inflated the catheter will then float into the right ventricle. Here the pressure will, of course, go up to around 20 ml. of mercury and the base of the curve will narrow out.

3. As the balloon floats the catheter through the pulmonary artery you will be able to know when it is past the pulmonary artery valve because the lowest deflection will be further from the bottom of the tracing due to valve closure. You will also note an extra upward deflection on the downward part of the curve. Finally, you will know when you are wedged when the total amplitude of the curve decreases markedly and the symmetry of the curve seems lost.

4. When this is achieved and the wedge pressure is obtained, pull back the catheter 2 cm. and deflate the balloon. The less you manipulate after that the longer the system will last (7 to 10 days if you are lucky).

5. If the patient has a disease in which there are indications for pacing (page 218) a "wide spectrum" catheter may be used, i.e., one that will give wedge pressure and cardiac output, and still have a stand-by pacer that will kick in at a certain heart rate. The future holds a fourth feature that will be a stand-by direct shock, given when--and if--ventricular fibrillation or cardiac arrest occurs. (Mirowski, Arch. Int. Med. 129, 1972).

With these remarks about the mechanics, what are the practical helps in patient management that we can get from balloon catheter directed monitoring? These are ever-increasing but the three main uses are 1) determining hypovolemia and monitoring fluid replacement; 2) determination of whether pulmonary congestion is due to heart failure or lung disease; and 3) the giving of precise prognostic and treatment information for management of cardiac function.

1. In a seriously ill patient who is suffering volume depletion--such as a burn --one can run in fluids at a rate as high as one liter an hour as long as the pulmonary artery pressure does not go over 20. When pulmonary artery pressure starts to rise from 0 to 5 (where it often is in hypovolemia) one can start to decrease the rate of fluid adminstration.

2. When pulmonary artery pressure is elevated or elevating and wedge pressure and cardiac output are staying normal and you know something is blocking circulation in the lung--this can lead us to early diagnosis of shock lung, pulmonary emboli, or fat emboli.

3. The combination of cardiac output and wedge pressure values allow you to get information that is of prognostic and therapeutic value regarding the failing heart, i.e., the stroke volume index and stroke work index. The stroke work should be at 30 or the heart is heading for trouble and in cardiogenic shock this figure should make one tend toward balloon pumping, angiography, and possible revascularization. Rather than use the numbers too arbitrarily while experience is being gained, the downward trend of the stroke work should be the ominous sign rather than the value itself.

HOW TO RECOGNIZE PULMONARY ARTERY CATHETER READINGS

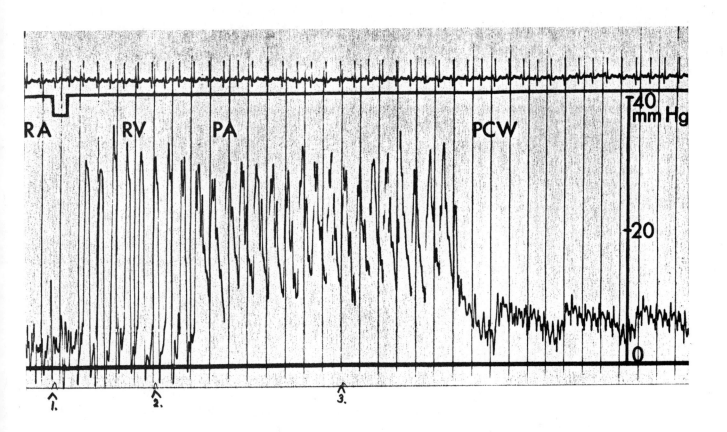

1. You usually know you are in the right auricle when you start to get pressure readings in a range of 1 to 5 ml. of mercury.

2. You are in the right ventricle when the amplitude of the curve increases markedly but the diastolic phase still goes to the base line.

3. You are in the pulmonary artery when the diastolic phase no longer meets the base line and when the downward part of the curve develops a notch.

4. You have wedged properly when the height of the curve decreases--its total amplitude decreases and the mean pressure is usually equal to the pulmonary artery diastolic pressure.

SHOCK LUNG - RESPIRATOR LUNG - WHITE LUNG

When this report comes back the patient will usually die. This syndrome occurs after a period of shock or time on the respirator and is evidenced by the abrupt appearance of a large, totally-white area on the chest x-ray. It is due to failure of the alveolar cells to function. Since it is so irreversible it is not unreasonable to use a "Prevention System" on patients who have prolonged shock or have been in a severe accident. The following Prevention System is the one used in our Burn Center and is unproven but reasonable.

SHOCK LUNG PREVENTION SYSTEM

1. All respirator patients are evaluated at least twice daily to get to the lowest pressure of PEEP (positive expiratory end pressure) and the lowest concentration of O_2 that will maintain an PaO_2 of 60.

2. Fifty ml. of 20% albumin is given I.V. every 6 hours to try to keep up pressure in the pulmonary capillaries.

3. Dilantin*, 100 mg., is given I.V. every 4 hours to inhibit the centroneurogenic factor in this syndrome.

TREATMENT SYSTEM FOR SHOCK

1. First rule out pulmonary edema as the cause of the picture, by digitalization and diuresis.

2. Use corticosteroids, decadron, 250 mg. to start, in 300 ml. of saline and then 50 mg. I.V. every 6 hours.

3. Dilantin*, 100 mg. I.V. every 6 hours. Check dilantin level after 4 doses. It should be in range of 10 to 20.

4. Use minimum of O_2 and PEEP to keep PaO_2 at 60 although you may try increasing PEEP rather than oxygen to get the alveolar spaces to open a bit.

5. Give as little fluid I.V. as you can to keep a urine output of 30 ml. an hour. When judging between kidney integrity and the white lung--let the kidneys go. Their damage will be more reversible and prolonged hemodialysis is better tolerated than prolonged ventilation.

6. Treat any infection to the maximum.

7. The shock lung patient who is not doing well is the prime candidate for the membrane oxygenator. Unfortunately we have not had enough experience with a membrane oxygenator as yet to give advice or direction as to its use. You can rest assured that by the time the next edition of this Manual rolls around the membrane oxygenator will be discussed in detail.

* Moss, Gerlad: The role of the central nervous system in shock: The centroneurogenic etiology of the respiratory distress syndrome. Critical Care Synposium, 3rd Ann. Mtg. of Soc. of Critical Care Medicine, Anaheim, Calif., 1974.

HYPOVOLEMIC SHOCK SYSTEM

The first step in treating any severe shock is to assume hypovolemia and run 250 ml. of plasmonate rapidly. This often will restore urine output and blood pressure. You may find you have been gradually getting behind in fluid due to excessive heat in the environment, vomiting, hyperventilation (which blows off a lot of water), diarrhea, simply not enough intake, or bleeding.

Hypovolemia is best treated with the aid of a pulmonary artery catheter, in that fluid can be rapidly replaced until the pulmonary artery systolic pressure goes up over five.

Blood volume should be adjusted to a baseline of at least 55 ml/kilo (page 79) search for bleeding should be made (page 101), and intake adjusted to 1.5 to 2 liters over output--adjusting Na to 140 and K to 4.

A ruptured aneurysm is, of course, a common cause of sudden unexplained hypovolemic shock and this should be ruled out with an ultrasound study of the abdomen. If it is in the thorax, the chest x-ray usually will point it out and immediate arrangements for cardiopulmonary bypass and repair should be made.

SYSTEM FOR TREATMENT OF GRAM-NEGATIVE (BACTERIAL) SHOCK

Criteria for institution of therapy for Gram-negative (bacterial) shock.
1. Blood pressure under 80

2. Pulse over 100

3. Temperature over 100.5° F. rectally

4. Stab count over 70

5. Positive blood culture for gram-negative bacilli. (Do NOT wait for this.)

6. No other apparent cause for shock.

DIAGNOSTIC CONTINGENCY ORDERS:
1. Blood culture--aerobic and anaerobic

2. Cultures of urine, stool, sputum, and any open wounds.

3. Serum amylase

4. Pulmonary artery catheter

5. Monitor heart

6. Chest x-ray, hourly urine output

7. If possible, culture for Herpes virus

8. Flat plate of abdomen to try to demonstrate free air.

ACTIVE CONTINGENCY ORDERS:
1. 500 cc. of plasmanate rapidly to rule out hypovolemic shock. If this restores blood pressure, you may relax a bit and perhaps concentrate on diagnosis before unloading full therapeutic barrage.

2. Ten gm. of chloramphenicol (chloromycetin) and 20 cc. of gamma globulin in 500 cc. of saline at 250 cc. per hour.

3. 150 mg. of gentamicin in 500 cc. of saline--100 cc. per hour--with $12\frac{1}{2}$ gm. of mannitol.

4. Methicillin, 10 gm. in 500 ml. D/5/W just in case a Staphylococcus is the culprit.

5. If the patient has leukemia, has been severely burned, or is on (or has been on) immunosuppressive drugs--give polymyxin B, 100 mg. in 500 ml. D/5/W.

6. Maintain arterial blood pressure at 70 with isuprel, 6 mg. in 300 ml. of saline microdrip. If this is not satisfactory, use 8 mg. of levophed* in 300 ml. of saline at rate to get blood pressure to 90 and run nipride at rate to decrease blood pressure 10--with the isuprel off. After the infusion rates are determined, run the levophed and nipride together.

7. Give 200 mg. of decadron or its equivalent, I.V. in 300 ml. of saline, and then 25 mg. I.V. every 8 hours. If the patient survives, this can be stopped after 24 hours.

8. Give piggyback, at rate of 100 ml. per hour, one liter of 50% glucose with 40 units of regular insulin, 60 mEq of KPO_4, and 500 mg. of vitamin C.

9. Give 8 ml. of cedilanid I.V.

10. If still NO blood pressure--consider aortic balloon pump augmentation--empirically, not on basis of pulmonary artery pressure.

11. Put down nasogastric tube.

12. If STILL NO blood pressure--search for operative lesion such as placentitis (abortion); obstructed ureter--do cytoscopy in bed if necessary; and, if possible, run a catheter around any internal obstructive stones. If you have obvious gynecological sepsis, explore and remove uterus. (I have seen patients in intractable gram-negative shock saved by removal of the uterus and by emergency surgery to relieve ureteral obstruction.)

In summary, then, gram-negative shock or septic shock is diagnosed by an unexplained low blood pressure, fever, high stab count, and, usually, inordinately good urine output.

It is cured by the sequential use of antibiotics, pressors, corticosteroids, aortic balloon pump, and surgery.

* Some physicians may prefer dopamine for this.

CARDIAC SHOCK SYSTEM, NAMELY, BLOOD PRESSURE UNDER 80 IN PRESENCE OF MYOCARDIAL INFARCTION

1. Place pulmonary artery catheter.

2. Start Cardiac Flowsheet (page 29).

3. Give plasmanate, 250 ml. an hour, until pulmonary artery pressure is over 20. If this maintains blood pressure of over 80--continue to monitor and observe.

4. Place indwelling catheter in bladder and record hourly urine output-- this will help you determine renal perfusion.

5. If plasmanate will NOT restore pressure--digitalize with cedilanid (page 196).

6. Monitor heart and use CONTINGENCIES FOR ARRHYTHMIAS (page 212-218).

7. Draw electrolytes and follow CONTINGENCY ORDERS indicated by them.

8. Start I.V.--500 ml. 50% glucose, 40 mEq KC1, 40 units of insulin, and 500 mg. of vitamin C per liter--and run at 100 ml. an hour, piggyback, in the pulmonary artery line.

9. If plasmanate, digitalization, and sugar, K, and insulin do NOT get blood pressure of 80 (60 is okay if urine output is over 20 ml. per hour), add insuprel, 3 mg. in 300 ml. D/5/W, and nipride, 50 mg. in 300 ml. D/5/W. Titer the isuprel by microdrip at rate to get systolic pressure at 90 and titer the nipride at rate to decrease blood pressure 10 ml. of mercury or at rate to decrease cardiac work index, then run them together.

10. If there is no response with isuprel, substitute norepinephrine, 8 mg. in 300 ml. D/5/W--or, if you prefer--dopamine, 50 mg. in 300 ml. D/5/W, in either case using microdrip. When you have established the dose of the pressor you are going to use, run it and the nipride together.

11. If the patient is STILL in shock while on plasmanate, digoxin, K, 50% glucose, insulin, isuprel, nipride, and norepinephrine--add 250 mg. of decadron I.V. in 300 ml. D/5/W to slow down release of proteolytic enzymes from dying cells.

12. If patient is STILL in shock while on plasmanate, digoxin, K, 50% glucose, insulin, isuprel, nipride, norepinephrine, and decadron--take him to the operating room and place an intra-aortic balloon pump and do an emergency angiogram. In a young patient I think the balloon should be started, even if getting emergency surgery done--that might be necessary--may pose logistics problems later.

13. If patient is stabilized on the pump, and if angiograms indicate possibility of repair, and if left ventricle has any life at all--put on bypass and repair the heart.

POTASSIUM CONTROL SYSTEM

Amount of potassium to be divided among the fluids to be given in the next 24 hours (adult). (KPO_4 instead of KCl when hyperalimentation is being used.)

Concentration

☐ 2.0 -- 2.9   200 mEq KCl

☐ 3.0 -- 3.4   180 "   "

☐ 3.5 -- 4.0   160 "   "

☐ 4.1 -- 4.5   150 "   "

☐ 4.6 -- 5.0   100 "   "

☐ 5.0 -- 5.5   75 "   "

☐   5.5   0

☐ Adjust every 12 hours. When this is used draw level every 12 hours and put in half the recommended daily dose in next 12 hours.

☐ Adjust every 4 hours. When this is used draw level every 4 hours and put in one-sixth of the recommended dose during next 4 hours.

☐ If BUN is greater than 25, half the suggested dose is to be used during the first two days until the need is established.

☐ Alternative K system. Replace K excretion in the 24-hour urine collection of the day before -- as long as level stays above 3.8.

NOTES

CARDIOGENIC SHOCK SYSTEM

Proof of efficacy of a CARDIOGENIC SHOCK SYSTEM will be hard to come by but each Unit's physicians should predetermine their opinions and actions regarding:

1. Placing of a pulmonary artery catheter and obtaining hemodynamic information.

2. Use of norepinephrine, lasix, corticosteroids, and digitalis.

3. Indications for angiography and surgery.

Most people with this condition die so an aggressive program is indicated. I use eight principles:

1. The use of enough fluid to get maximum cardiac output by Starling's law, i.e., push fluids to the pulmonary artery pressures that give maximum cardiac output.

2. Ionotropic agents to the point that they start to increase heart work.

3. Peripheral vascular dilatation to the point that pressors will still get perfusion.

4. Corticosteroids to slow down the vicious cycle of dying by stabilizing the lysosomes of the dying cells in the heart and elsewhere (decadron, 50 mg. q. 6 hours).

5. Enough lasix to reduce myocardial depressant factor.

6. Standby rhythm control by a standby pacer and lidocaine Contingency Orders.

7. Aortic balloon pump if necessary to increase output and decrease after load.

8. Angiography and surgery if with a high pulmonary artery pressure, digitalis, and pressors the work is increasing and the cardiac output is not enough to effect perfusion.

SYSTEM FOR MANAGING ANAPHYLACTIC SHOCK

The tipoff regarding anaphylactic shock is the tremendous shortness of breath and dyspnea that is inordinate for this physical finding. Secondly, there is always a history of receiving a medication within the past several hours.

Remember, the medication could have been taken by mouth as well as by injection. The most common cause at present is probably penicillin and hydrodiuril, but almost any medication can cause it. Aspirin, even a single aspirin, can do this, and insect bites are also common causes. Whatever the cause, adrenalin is the treatment of choice and it should be given intravenously (4 ml. of a 1:10,000 dilution)--two ampules--and it should be repeated in 5 minutes. In addition, O_2 should be given and, if the patient still seems to be choking, put down an endo-tracheal tube and use PEEP if necessary to get the ApO_2 over 50.

If the patient does not respond rapidly, give 100 mg. of decadron in 300 ml. of saline by rapid drip as well. The issue of life and death from anaphylactic shock is usually decided rapidly and adrenalin and corticosteroids and forcing oxygen through the alviolar cells are the sine qua nons of therapy.

SINGLE LIFE LINE INTRAVENOUS SUPPORT SYSTEM

There are numerous patients in Critical Care Units in whom it is only humane to draw off all blood and administer all medications through a single intravenous line, which is in the vena cava. Nursing Services and Pharmacies, and correctly so, have devised numerous "No, no"s regarding mixing medications and using lines for multiple uses. However, the admonitions have to be ignored in situations where the patient is being made to suffer unduly by blood-drawing, extra I.V. lines, and extra I.M. injections. Therefore, I hope the physicians who treat this type of patient will agree with me that this type of patient should be supported with a single life line, and that they will insist that rules regarding mixing of medications and infusions be lifted for those patients. When the single line intravenous support system is ordered, then the nurse is to be instructed to piggyback (put I.V. needle in the main line) medications and to draw all blood off the vena cava line.

All blood transfusions are to be given this way also. This will often cause hyperalimentation to be interrupted while blood or plasmanate is given, and, in this case, 50% glucose may have to be injected every two hours while this is being done. It will mean that intralipid is piggybacked into the line as near the clavicle as possible, and that, if the mixtures are clearly incompatible, saline may be run for short periods while certain infusions are piggybacked. However, with careful daily planning, patients can be maintained completely on a single subclavian line and thus be spared all blood letting and I.M. injections during the acutely painful phase of their illness.

Patients such as these also should have an arterial line placed, since multiple blood gas determinations are often necessary and multiple femoral sticks are painful as well as dangerous. In this case the routine blood determinations can also be drawn off the femoral line. If the patient is on dialysis, whenever possible a shunt with a spigot for drawing blood should be placed, as drawing blood from this will often save patients much torture that would result if other methods of monitoring were used.

DIRECTIONS FOR DRAWING BLOOD FROM A SUBCLAVIAN LINE

Supplies: 1 -- 20 cc. syringe.

1 -- 12 cc. syringe with 10 cc. saline.

Necessary specimen tubes for:
Blood gases   -- 3 cc. heparinized syringe
Glucose   -- Green-topped tube
K   -- Green-topped tube
Hematocrit & hemoglobin (H & H)   -- Purple-topped tube

Procedure:

A. Drawing off 20 cc.s of blood:
   1. Disconnect adaptor of subclavian line from regular administration set.

   2. Connect tip of 20 cc. syringe to adaptor of subclavian line. Draw off 20 cc. of blood.   Then disconnect 20 cc. syringe from adaptor.

B. Obtaining necessary specimens:
   1. Blood gases -- a 3 cc. heparinized syringe is needed. Place syringe in ice after blood sample is obtained.

   2. For glucose (green-topped tube), K (green-topped tube), and H & H purple-topped tube) a Multi-Sample Adaptor is needed.
       (If a Multi-Sample Adaptor is not available, the blood can be transferred to the necessary tubes by using a 12 cc. syringe and a needle.)

C. After specimens are obtained:
   1. If the specimens are drawn in less than one minute, the initial 20 cc. of blood may be given back through the subclavian line.

   2. If the time lapse was more than one minute, discard the 20 cc. of blood.

   3. Then--flush the line with 10 cc. of saline.

   4. Reconnect the administration set to the adaptor of the subclavian line.

PROCEDURE FOR DRAWING BLOOD FROM A SUBCLAVIAN LINE IF SUPPORT DRUGS ARE RUNNING

Supplies: 1 -- 20 cc. syringe.

1 -- 12 cc. syringe filled with 10 cc. of saline.

Necessary specimen tubes.

Procedure:

1. Take clean 20 cc. syringe and proceed to draw off 20 cc. of blood.

2. Take necessary containers to draw blood for specimens.

3. Give back original 20 cc. of blood IF procedure was completed in less than one minute.

4. Flush the subclavian line with 10 cc. of saline.

5. Give back the support drug fluid. (This prevents giving a bolus of support drug medication.)

6. Reconnect administration set to the adaptor of the subclavian line.

HYPERALIMENTATION SYSTEM

We are inclined to agree with Dr. Dudrick, the young father of hyperalimentation, that 40 per cent of hospitalized patients could benefit from the modality. Burns, postoperative patients, patients on dialysis, patients receiving cancer chemotherapy, and patients with colitis are particularly apt to benefit.

In my experience two modifications make the use of hyperalimentation easy and safe. The first is the addition of small doses of antibiotics to the solution to keep it sterile, and the second is to give the solution through a regular intravenous line without a filter. (Since the solution is kept sterile by the antibiotics there is no need for the filter, which slows down administration markedly.) In addition, potassium, insulin, phosphate, and magnesium should be added to the solution.

The release of intralipid has added fat to the protein and sugar in freamine and this should be added to the program, using the following system.

Start with one liter of hyperalimentation and 250 ml. of intralipid and work up to four liters of hyperalimentation and one liter of intralipid in a cachetic patient.

HYPERALIMENTATION ORDER SHEET

1. Give _____ liters of freamine solution, modified by the addition of the following:
    a. Regular insulin--40 units.
    b. KPO_4 -- 40 mEq.
    c. Amphotericin B, one mg. (kills fungus).
    d. Polymyxin B, one mg. (kills Pseudomonas).
    e. Gentamicin, one mg. (kills Staphylococcus and Klebsiella).

2. Give _____ ml. of intralipid daily (if piggyback in subclavian, put 10 cm. from place where line enters the subclavian region).

3. Give daily--B_{12}, 1000 ug. I.V. and folic acid, one mg. I.V., into tubing.

4. Give 10 cc. of calcium gluconate every 8 hours--IF BUN normal.

5. Determine and record daily intake, daily output, calories, blood sugar, BUN daily; serum osmolality, weight, hemoglobin, WBC, Ca, K, Na, and triglycerides (if one intralipid) three times a week; and zinc, magnesium, and blood ammonia once a week.

6. Edecrin, 50 mg., if intake is greater than 4 liters over output, or there is a 3 lb. weight gain in a day.

7. First 2 days check blood sugar 3 times a day and use following schedule:

Blood Sugar	Regular Insulin
500	40 -- repeat in 2 hours (same schedule)
400 -- 500	30 -- repeat in 4 hours
300 -- 399	25 -- repeat in 8 hours
200 -- 299	10 -- repeat in 8 hours

8. If hypoglycemic--decrease insulin in hyperalimentation. (Children often need none added).

9. After first few days check urine sugar 4 times a day and, if 4+, give 20 units of regular insulin and check in 2 hours. Give 20 units of regular insulin each time urine shows 4+.

10. If hemoglobin under 10--give a unit of cell mass (page 101).

11. If WBC has unexpected rise--get chest x-ray, liver scan, look in eye grounds (for embolic spots), and blood culture. Culture I.V. fluid and change line if no overt cause of the rise.

12. If BUN over 30--adjust amount of hyperalimentation solution to keep BUN stable.

13. If serum ammonia over 8--discontinue hyperalimentation. The patient cannot handle the protein.

14. If the serum osmolality is over 350--discontinue the hyperalimentation. You may be getting into hyperosmolality syndrome because the cells cannot metabolize the excess load.

15. If the Na is over 150, see page 123. Usually you can correct this with a few extra liters of D/5/W.

16. If K is more than 5 or less than 4--adjust K in the solution or, if patient is on digitalis, correct with 60 mg. of KPO_4 by volutrol in 200 ml. of saline over 2 hours.

17. If triglycerides rise more than 50--reduce quantity of intralipid.

18. If magnesium is 1.4--increase magnesium sulfate in the hyperalimentation, but if magnesium is 1.9--decrease magnesium sulfate in the hyperalimentation.

19. If zinc is 1--if possible augment hyperalimentation by 4 to 6 zincate tablets by mouth or nasogastric tube.

20. If calcium (page 132) is over 10--discontinue calcium gluconate, but if it is less than 6--increase calcium gluconate to every 4 hours until level is above 8.

21. Weight--if over 3 lb. weight gain in 24 hours--give edecrin, 50 mg. I.V. If not excellent response--discontinue the hyperalimentation.

SYSTEM FOR FEVER OF UNKNOWN ETIOLOGY SYSTEM

Fever that is unexplainable can almost always be explained by the following System that rules out infection, neoplasm, autoimmunity, metabolism as the cause. Things on the physical exam that are the most helpful are heart murmurs, biopsied lymph nodes, palpable organs, skin lesions such as petechiae, and joint swellings. However, if I had only one modality with which to diagnose F.U.O., I would choose the taking of a careful history.

LABORATORY WORKUP OF A F.U.O.:

Culture -- Blood, urine, sputum, stool, spinal fluid, and any drainage -- aerobically and anaerobically.

Biopsy and Culture -- Lymph node, scalene if necessary, and liver.

Scan-Gallium -- Total body -- liver, spleen, pancreas, bones, and lungs.

X-ray -- Stomach, small bowel, kidneys, colon, gallbladder, and bones.

Serology -- Sabin dye test; heterophile; cold agglutinins; Epstein-Barr; thyroid; Proteus, o-- 19O; CEA titer; Brucella agglutinins; tularemia agglutinins; complement fixation for leptospirosis, blastomycosis, histoplasmosis, coccidioidomycosis, Psittocosis influenza mycoplasma; antinuclear antibodies; and rheumatoid factor.

Liver function -- LDH, SGOT, and Na.

Cardiac function -- EKG, C reactive protein, and antistreptolysin titer.

Lumbar puncture -- India ink, cell block, culture for fungi, Tbc, and anaerobes

Urine -- etiocholanalone level, midstream culture, cellular elements, Bence-Jones protein.

Quantitative immunoglobulins - IgA, IgM, IgG

Complement level

Ultrasound of abdomen for lymph nodes

If all of these tests are normal (do them sequentially at a rate dictated by the velocity of the patient's illness), surgical exploration usually is necessary to diagnose the lymphoma or tuberculosis that may be present. If you are to explore always take out the spleen and get biopsies of the liver, kidneys, muscles, skin, and lymph nodes. Culture the material as well as prepare it histologically and, if possible, have electron microscopy done on the kidneys, muscle, and liver.

NOTES

PULMONARY EMBOLISM SYSTEM

1. Give atropine I.V., 0.75 mg. (1/100 grain).

2. Give isuprel 3 mg. in 300 ml. of saline at rate to keep blood pressure at 100.

3. Start respirator as indicated by blood gases. If patient does NOT stabilize, do pulmonary angiogram and have any large embolus removed surgically.

4. If angiograms and surgery are not feasible, give heparin, 5000 units I.V. (50 mg.) every 4 hours--checking either clotting time or recal time before every fourth dose.

5. Do pelvic and leg angiograms to try to localize source of embolus and tie off or screen vena cava if indicated. A repeat pulmonary embolus from an unknown source usually is a good indication for tying off the vena cava.

6. As the patient gets better take her off birth control pills and check her or him for carcinoma of the pancreas or lung, for lupus erythematosus, and for hypercoagulability (clot stretch test).

7. Keep on heparin for two weeks and coumadin for six weeks.

CHECK SHEET FOR PULMONARY EMBOLUS

☐ Atropine

☐ Isuprel--control blood pressure

☐ Angiograms -- pulmonary

☐ . . . . . . -- legs

☐ . . . . . . -- pelvis

☐ Consider surgery

☐ Rule out -- lupus

☐ . . . . . -- birth control pill

☐ . . . . . -- occult carcinoma

SYSTEM FOR PREVENTION OF FAT EMBOLISM

This sytem should be invoked when ever a large bone fracture occurs in a young person and whenever there are three significant fractures in any patient.

DAILY DIAGNOSTIC TESTS:

1. Arterial blood gases.

2. Chest x-ray.

3. Urine for fat globules.

ACTIVE THERAPY:

1. When and if either the blood gases start to indicate a problem or the chest x-ray shows unexplained infiltration -- pulmonary artery monitoring should be started and an arterial line placed. Lung function should be kept as normal as possible by the reaction to the blood gases and pulmonary artery pressures (pages 61, 69, 87).

2. Give decadron, 100 mg. I.V. in 300 ml. of saline, then 50 mg. every 6 hours.

3. Invoke the shock lung preventive program given on page 172.

DRUG FAIL -- SAFE SYSTEMS

All drugs ordered are to be checked by the ward secretary or pharmacy representative in the HOSPITAL FORMULARY and possible toxicities noted on a Toxicity Alert Flowsheet, along with suggested toxicity monitoring. I have concluded that drug incompatibility problems are best checked, computerwise if possible, in the Pharmacy itself, where each patient's drug profile should be scanned each day, one way or another, for drug incompatibilities.

See example (page 195) of Drug Alert Flowsheet, which should be a part of the patient's chart. Routine Drug Alerts can be developed by each Unit.

DRUGS THAT CAUSE ANEMIA AND HOW THEY DO IT

The first step is to discontinue them if the patient is anemic--then:
a. Get Coombs' test.
b. Get test for glucose 6-phosphate dehydrogenase deficiency if patient is receiving drugs under category #4 or #5.

c. Get reticulocyte count.

1. DRUGS THAT CAUSE MEGALOBLASTIC ANEMIA (MCV over 100):
   a. Diphenylhydantoin (dilantin)   d. Arsenic
   b. Oral contraceptive agents   e. Barbiturates
   c. Methotrexate

2. DRUGS THAT CAUSE ANEMIA BY INTERFERING WITH HEMESYNTHESIS INH (to prevent this, always give drug with PYRIDOXINE).

3. DRUGS THAT ARE TOXIC TO THE BONE MARROW:
   a. Chloramphenicol (chloromycetin)
   b. Mephenytoin (mesantoin--used for epilepsy)
   c. Phenylbutazone (butazolidin)
   d. Gold salts
   e. Amphotericin B (fungizone, mystecline)
   f. Phenothiazine

4. DRUGS THAT CAUSE BLEEDING: Aspirin compounds of all kinds.

5. DRUGS THAT CAUSE IMMUNE HEMOLYTIC ANEMIA (Coombs test and high reticulocyte count establish this):
   a. Methyldopa
   b. Penicillin
   c. Cephalothin

6. DRUGS THAT CAUSE NONIMMUNE HEMOLYTIC ANEMIA (Get glucose-6-phosphate dehydrogenase deficiency):
   a. Primaquine and related antimalarials
   b. Sulfonamides
   c. Sulfones (dapsone, etc.)
   d. Nitrofurans
   e. Salicylates
   f. Phenacetin
   g. Dimercaprol (BAL)
   h. Methylene blue
   i. Naphthalene (moth balls)
   j. Probenacid
   k. Chloramphenicol
   l. Menadione (K_3), Kappadione, Synkayvite

DRUGS THAT INCREASE PROTHROMBIN TIME

ACETOMINOPHEN

ACETOHEXAMIDE

ACETYLSALICYLIC ACID (large doses)

AMINOSALICYLIC ACID

ASPARAGINASE

CATHARTICS

CHLORAMPHENICOL

CHLORDIAZEPOXIDE

CHLORPROMAZINE

CHLORPROPAMIDE

CHLORTETRACYCLINE

CHOLESTRAMINE

CREOMYCIN

CYCLOPHOSPHAMIDE

DEMECLOCYCLINE

DOXYCYCLINE

HALOTHANE

KANAMYCIN

LAXATIVES

MEPAZINE

MERCAPTOPURINE

METHOTREXATE

METHYLTESTOSTERONE

MINERAL OIL

NEOMYCIN

NIACIN

ORAL CONTRACEPTIVES

PROCHLORPERAZINE

PROMAZINE

PYRAZINAMIDE

QUINIDINE

QUININE

STREPTOMYCIN

SUCCINYLSULFATHIAZOLE

SULFAMETHOZAZOLE

SULFACHLORPYRIDAZINE

SUFFISOXAZOLE

TETRACYCLINE

THIAZIDES

TOLAZAMIDE

TOLBUTAMIDE

TRIFLUOPERAZINE

TYPES OF TOXICITIES TO BE EXPECTED FROM VARIOUS DRUGS

Here's a list of common drug reactions and the drugs that cause them;

Anemia

chloramphenicol
chloroquine
gold salts
hydantoins
mephenytoin
methyldopa
phenothiazines
phenylbutazone
primidone
quinacrine
sulfonamides
thiouracils
trimethadione

Asthma

antihistamines
dextran
penicillin
pollen extracts
reserpine
salicylates
serum

Bullous Eruptions

antibiotics
bromides
hydantoins
insulin
iodides
penicillins
phenothiazines
sulfonamides

Eczematous Dermatitis

antibiotics
antihistamines
arsenicals
bromides
chloral hydrate
iodides
mercurials
PAS
penicillin
quinacrine
streptomycin
sulfonamides

Eosinophilia

ACTH
isoniazid
kanamycin
phenothiazines
penicillin
streptomycin

Erythema Multiforme-like Eruptions

antibiotics
barbiturates
bromides
gold salts
iodides
meprobamate
penicillin
phenacetin
phenolphthalein
salicylates
sulfonamides

Erythema Nodosum

bromides
iodides
salicylates
sulfonamides

Exanthematous Eruptions

antibiotics
barbiturates
belladonna
bromides
chloroquine
diethylstilbestrol
gold salts
hydantoins
mercurials
PAS
penicillin
phenothiazines
quinacrine
quinidine
reserpine
salicylates
serums & organ
  extracts
sulfonamides
thiouracils

Exfoliative Dermatitis

acetazolamide
barbiturates
chloroquine
gold salts
hydantoins
iodides
mercurials
penicillin
phenothiazines
phenylbutazone
quinacrine
sulfonamides

Fever

isoniazid
mercurials
nitrofurantoins
penicillin
procainamide
quinidine
sulfonamides

Fixed Eruptions

acetophenetidin
barbiturates

gold salts
iodides
phenolphthalein
quinacrine
quinidine
sulfonamides

Granulocytopenia

acetazolamide
ACTH
aminopyrine
antihistamines
arsenicals
chloramphenicol
chloroquine
cinophen
gold salts
hydantoins
hydralazine
novobiocin
phenacetin
phenothiazines
phenurone
phenylbutazone
procainamide
salicylates
streptomycin
sulfonamides
sulfonylureas
tetracyclines
thiazides
thiouracils

Hepatic Damage

adrenergic hormones
anabolic agents
anesthetics
antimalarials
barbiturates
chlorothiazide
chlorpromazine
erythromycin
estrogens
gold salts
hydantoins
ilosone
isoniazid
novobiocin
PAS
phenothiazines
phenurone
phenylbutazone
probenecid
sulfonamides
sulfonylureas
thiouracils
triacetyloleandomycin

Löffler-like Syndrome

mercurials
nitrofurantoins
PAS

Nephritis and/or Nephrosis

acetazolamide
amphotericin B
antibiotics
cycloserine
gold salts
iodides
mercurials
paramethadione
phenacetin
phenylbutazone
probenecid
serums
sulfonamides
sulfonylureas
thiazides
trimethadione

Periarteritis Nodosa

hydantoins
iodides
mercurials
penicillin
phenylbutazone
serums
sulfonamides
thiouracils

Photosensitivity

dimethylchlor-
  tetracycline
quinidine
sulfonamides
thiazides

Purpura, Nonthrombocytopenic

barbiturates
gold salts
heparin
isoniazid
penicillin
phenacetin
phenothiazines
quinidine
sulfonamides

Purpura, Thrombocytopenic

chloramphenicol
penicillin
quinidine
quinine
sulfonamides

Serum-like Sickness

antibiotics
antihistamines
barbiturates
heparin

hydantoins
hydralazine
mercurials
organ extracts
penicillin
procainamide
quinidine
salicylates
serums
streptomycin
sulfonamides
thiouracils
vaccines

Shock

ACTH
anesthetics, local
antibiotics
BSP
chymotrypsin
dehydrocholic acid
dextran
diphenhydramine
DPT
folic acid (IV)
gamma globulin
heparin
iodides
meperidine
meprobamate
mercurials
nicotinic acid
nitrofurantoin
organ extracts
oxytocin
penicillins
pollen extracts
salicylates
sedative hypnotics
serums
sulfonamides
tetanus toxoid
thiamine
vaccines

SLE-like Picture

hydantoins
hydralazine
penicillin
procainamide
sulfonamides
thiazides.

Urticaria

ACTH
antibiotics
insulin
liver extracts
penicillin
pollen extracts
serums
streptomycin
sulfonamides

DRUG ALERT FLOWSHEET

DRUG	TARGET ORGAN	MONITORING TEST	CONTINGENCY ORDER
Chloramphenicol	Bone marrow	Daily retic	D.C. if 2 days running > .2
Aminoglycosides: Antibiotics - Tobramycin Streptomycin Neomycin	Kidneys Hearing	Daily BUN level M.W.F. Ask daily about hearing	Halve dose if BUN up 5 from previous day or level > 5. D.C. if level > 8 or divide daily dose by serum creatinine level
Digoxin	Arrhythmia Nausea	EKG - K - BUN	Hold if K under 3.6. Halve dose if BUN > 30 (See page 113 EKG)
Sodium Nitroprusside	Cyanide intoxication Hypotension	Cyanide levels Blood pressure	D.C. if levels > 10 Slow rate if blood pressure 65
Carbenicillin	Bleeding	BUN Prothrombin time	Halve dose if BUN up 5 With large doses precede dose c̄ 25 mg. mephyton
Polymyxin B	Renal Paralysis	BUN Serum calcium	Halve dose if BUN up > 5 from previous day Precede I.V. administration c̄ 10 ml. calcium gluconate
Cytoxan	Bone marrow	CBC & platelets M.F.W.	HOLD if WBC < 4000 or platelets <100,000
Edecrin	Hearing	BUN Ask about hearing	Halve dose if BUN > 30 HOLD if hearing difficulty
Aldomet	Immune anemia Fever	Hemoglobin weekly Coombs' test monthly Check temperature	D.C. if anemia develops or patient feverish
Quinidine	Hearing Platelets	Level of M.W.F. Platelet level weekly	Decrease dose if level > 8

DIGITALIS SYSTEM

The ready availability of digoxin levels make it mandatory that acutely ill patients who are receiving digitalis have a level drawn each day and that the daily dose be predicated on that level.

The other variables to be considered are:

1. Individual reactions (some patients can become toxic with digitalis at levels far under the suggested range of 1.5 to 2.5).

2. Age--elderly people generally need a smaller dose.

3. Weight--the usual dose to maintain a digoxin level of around 1.8 to 2 is 0.25 to 0.50 mg. of digoxin per day. Patients under 100 lbs. usually need one-half this dose, but obese individuals cannot be arbitrarily increased and must be managed on the basis of levels. If weight is under 50 lbs. give 1/4 the dose.

4. Potassium level--the K level should be adjusted to 4 by volutrol before the daily digoxin dosage is administered (see K System--pages 127, 129).

5. Calcium--Calcium should NOT be administered within 2 hours before or after digoxin. Patients who are hypercalcemic (Over 10) should be given one-half the dose.

6. Kidney function--patients with elevated BUN tend to have high levels and if BUN is over 25 the schedule should be given at half dose.

7. Recent myocardial patients--these patients should be given digitalis very gingerly and I favor treating mild failure with diuretics. If they are digitalized I do it with lidocaine running or with quinidine beforehand.

DIGITALIZATION

1. If patient is fibrillating give 0.75 to 0.25 mg. of digoxin every 4 hours until apical rate is between 60 and 80.

2. Patient not fibrillating--give 0.75 mg. of digoxin (I.V. or oral) then follow this schedule based on daily digoxin levels:

Digoxin Level *	Dose of Digoxin	
2.5	0	
2.0 -- 2.5	0.125	Have K 4 or over.
1.6 -- 1.9	0.25	Halve dose if BUN over 25
1.0 -- 1.5	0.50	or age over 65
1.0	0.75	

* NOTE - There are for some reason particularly wide differences in "normal" digoxin levels in various laboratories - so check the levels with your laboratory.

Adjust this schedule to maintain level at around 2. If--in 2 days--level is not rising, INCREASE the dose schedule one notch, i.e., 2.0 -- 2.5 to 0.25, etc.

If BUN is up 5 from day before--halve the dose.

If EKG shows superventricular tachycardia or PVC -- hold for orders.

If rate under 65--hold dose.

DIGITALIZATION IN CHILDREN

Age	Dose for Total Digitalization
< one month	35 ug/kilo (micrograms NOT milligrams)
one month to 10 years	40 ug/kilo

Give one-half dose STAT and one-half in 4 hours. Titrate each child's level to 2 by starting with one-fourth the digitalization dose daily and adjusting by the daily level. Babies under three usually need 0.1 or 0.05 mg/day for maintenance.

NOTES

REMARKS ABOUT INTRA-AORTIC BALLOON PUMPING SYSTEM

This simple device helps the heart along by lowering aortic pressure prior to left ventricular ejection so more blood gets out of the heart, and heightening it during diastole so that more oxygenated blood goes into the coronary and renal arteries.

Its use in all kinds of pump failure, and particularly in allowing emergency surgery in patients in acute cardiogenic shock, is well documented (page 243); therefore it will be used in an increasing number of Critical Care Units. Its absolute contraindications are: aortic insufficiency and dissecting aneurisms.

The manuals that come with the machines are excellent and need not be paraphrased here. The fundamental adjustment of the balloon counterpulsation pump is that of triggering the balloon inflation to occur just after the close of the aortic valve. The R wave on the EKG is used as a reference point and the crucial setting is the inflate timing control, which must be adjusted to show inflation at between the 20 to 70 percent interval between two R waves. Once the balloon pump has been placed this is usually the only control that must be adjusted, with the remainder of the controls being warning devices and weaning devices. About a 4-hour orientation course with observation should be adequate to instruct a critical care nurse in the monitoring of a balloon counterpulsation device as long as there is always good communication with the bioengineer and the responsible physician of the Unit.

The pump can be shut off for 4 to 6 hours and pumping then reinstituted (for things like hyperbaric oxygen therapy),but this, of course, incurs a calculated risk of emboli forming (page 232).

COUMADIN ANTICOAGULATION SYSTEM

If you feel the patient should be anticoagulated, either to prevent or to treat an embolic phenomenon, use the following system:

Get base line prothrombin time and if it is 12 or under, give 20 mg. of coumadin and then order daily prothrombin times and follow the schedule below:

Dosage of Coumadin	Prothrombin Time in Seconds
15 mg.	12 or under
$12\frac{1}{2}$ mg.	13 -- 15
10 mg.	16 -- 17
$7\frac{1}{2}$ mg.	18 -- 20
5 mg.	21 -- 22
$2\frac{1}{2}$ mg.	23 -- 24
0	over 24

You will note this is self-correcting. If you find the time goes over 24 seconds too often, decrease each dose by $2\frac{1}{2}$ mg.

Check pages following for drugs that potentiate coumadin, and if patient is receiving one of these--decrease each suggested dose of coumadin by $2\frac{1}{2}$ mg. until you have determined the correct dose to keep level at between 18 to 24 seconds.

DRUGS THAT TEND TO POTENTIATE COUMADIN ANTICOAGULANTS
(PROTHROMBIN TIME INCREASED)

BY COMPETING WITH ALBUMIN BINDING SITES:

CHLORAL HYDRATE

CLOFIBRATE

DIAZOXIDE

ETHACRYNIC ACID

INDOMETHACIN

MEFENAMIC ACID

NALIDIXIC ACID

OXYPHENBUTAZONE

PHENYLBUTAZONE

PROBENECID

SULFONAMIDES

TRICLOFOS

BY INHIBITING COUMADIN METABOLISM:

ANABOLIC STEROIDS

CHLORAMPHENICOL

CYCLOPHOSPHAMIDE

DEXTROTHYROXINE

L-ASPARAGINASE

MERCAPTOPURINE

MITHRAMYCIN

PHENYREMIDOL

PROPYLTHIOURACIL

DRUGS THAT TEND TO INHIBIT COUMADIN ANTICOAGULANTS

(PROTHROMBIN TIME DECREASED)

BY ENHANCING COUMADIN METABOLISM:

BARBITURATES	GLUTETHEMIDE
CARBAMAZEPINE	GRISEOFULVIN
CHLOROBUTANOL	ORPHENADRINE
CORTICOTROPIN	TOLBUTAMIDE
ETHCHLORMYNOL	VITAMIN K

BY DECREASING COUMADIN ABSORPTION:

CHOLESTYRAMINE	VITAMIN A (large doses)

ANTICOAGULATION SYSTEM WITH HEPARIN

1. Give 5000 units* of heparin every 6 hours.

2. On alternate days get recal time or Lee-White clotting time just <u>before</u> a dose of heparin and 20 minutes <u>after</u> a dose of heparin. In this way you will be sure to know whether you are achieving therapeutic levels (Lee-White time--over 12 seconds; recal time--over 6 seconds). When you get the level just <u>before</u> the dose it will tell you are giving too much heparin, in which case <u>the dose</u> can be reduced; or, if the Lee-White time stays up, protamine, 50 mg. I.V., can be given.

* This dose is a minimum - your Unit may want to quadruple it.

SYSTEM FOR EMERGENCY SEARCH FOR BLEEDING DIATHESIS*

1. Determine if there is a previous history of bleeding from dental work or venipunctures. If the answer is YES it may be a sign of:

    a. Mild hemophilia
    b. Christmas disease
    c. von Willebrand's disease
    d. Familial thrombocytopathy

2. Is bleeding multifocal? If the answer is YES it suggests a generalized problem.

3. Order bleeding diathesis screening panel (page 43). (Negotiate this beforehand with your Clinical Laboratory.)

    a. Platelet count ⎫
    b. Bleeding time ⎬ To test platelet function
    c. Prothrombin time--if normal excludes disseminating intravascular coagulation
    d. Partial thromboplastin time (isolated abnormality equals hemophilia A or Christmas disease)
    e. Thrombin time (best for severe hypofibrinogenia)
    f. Test for circulating heparin in plasma
    g. Test for indigenous circulating anticoagulant
    h. Test for fibrin split products (elevated in D.I.C.)
    i. Blood smear to search for red cell fragments and to check platelet count
    j. Clot solubility test (checks for factor VIII deficiency)

* Based on an article by Peter Levine, Arch. Int. Med., Sept., 1972

SYSTEM FOR DEALING WITH A POTENTIALLY COMPROMISED HOST

Increasingly patients in Critical Care Units will fall into the category of <u>compromised hosts.</u> These patients must be identified and given special treatment. They deserve MORE attention rather than less. This is the reason we suggest that isolation be reserved for <u>very</u> special cases and that most cases be treated with prophylactic antibiotics rather than isolation.

PROPHYLACTIC SYSTEM FOR PATIENTS WHO HAVE COMPROMISED RESISTANCE

1. Identify patient who falls into this group by checking diagnosis against Table 1

2. Keep Compromised Host Flowsheet up-to-date

3. Use one line technique (page 181)   and do NOT give intramuscular or subcutaneous injections to these patients

4. Complete bath with pHisoHex--daily

5. Gentamicin ointment to external nares--once daily

6. Immune panel--weekly:
   a. Quantitative immunoglobulins
   b. T-cell percentage
   c. M.I.F.
   d. Total complement
   e. Complement #3
   f. WBC

7. Cultures of nose, throat, stool, urine, and blood-weekly

8. Patients with WBC under 2500, patients with acute leukemia, or patients on Imuran:
   a. Oxacillin, 0.5 gm. by mouth 3 times a day
   b. Flucytosine, 500 mg. by mouth 4 times a day

9. Multivalent vaccine - weekly

10. Transfer factor every 2 weeks

11. Unexplained fever must be completely ruled out by the Immunodepressed Fever of Unknown Origin Check Sheet (page 187). Do all of the tests in the <u>middle</u> column until a diagnosis is made.

If you have a potentially salvagable patient who is immunosuppressed and dying of overwhelming sepsis, you may want to use the program I have used on occasion: (page 232).

Chloramphenicol   8 grams

Gentamycin   150 mgm

Methicillin   8 grams

Polymyxin B   150 mgm

Cytosine Arabinoside   80 mgm

Pentimamide   40 mgm I. M. - q 6 hours

Decadron   100 mgm

COMPROMISED HOSTS IN CRITICAL CARE UNIT

1. Organ transplants

2. Acute leukemics under chemotherapy

3. Severe burns

4. Childhood or adult granulomatous disease

5. After fourth day on respirator

6. Cancer under x-ray and chemotherapy

7. Autoimmune diseases - L.E., dermatomyositis, etc.

8. Agranulocytosis from whatever cause

9. Patients on high doses of corticosteroids

10. Hodgkin's disease under multiple therapy

11. Thymic aplasia

12. Others to be added by Critical Care Committee:

    a.

    b.

    c.

    d.

DIAGNOSTIC AND THERAPEUTIC CHECK SHEET FOR IMMUNODEPRESSED PATIENT WITH UNEXPLAINED FEVER OR UNEXPLAINED PULMONARY LESION

POSSIBLE DISEASE	DIAGNOSTIC TESTS	THERAPY
Pneumocystis Carinii	Lung biopsy if platelets over 80 M Bronchial brush Transtracheal aspiration (stain c̄ methenamine silver)	Penicillin Flagyl
Salmonella	Culture	Chloramphenicol
Toxoplasmosis	Sabin dye test Lymph node biopsy	Daraprim (Pyri-methamine) 25 mg/day. Sulfadiazone and gamma globulin
Herpes Simplex A & B	Culture on cell lines Complement fixation	Cytosine arabinoside OR Idoxiuridine and gamma globulin and transfer factor
Cytomegalic inclusion body disease	Culture on cell lines Stain urine and look especially for culture urine on cell lines	Cytosine arabinoside and gamma globulin and transfer factor
Varicella (chickenpox Herpes Zoster)	Culture on cell lines Good history of exposure Characteristic skin lesions	Cytosine arabinoside gamma globulin transfer factor
Listeria	Intracellular Gram + bacilli in CNS	Penicillin
Tuberculosis	Gastrics (YES-gastrics) ZN smear	3-drug Rx -- strep-tomycin, INH, PAS, ethambutal, Rifampin

SYSTEM FOR HANDLING DIABETIC COMA AND/OR DIABETIC HYPERGLYCEMIA, HYPEROSMOLALITY, AND LACTIC ACIDOSIS

1. Normalize blood sugar with insulin:

BLOOD SUGAR LEVEL	REGULAR INSULIN
600	Regular insulin,* 50 units every 90 minutes, given subcutaneously (I.V. if the patient is in shock or in extremis), until blood sugar level is lower than time before--then 35 units per 90 minutes until blood sugar level is under 600.
450-599	Regular insulin, 35 units every 90 minutes, given subcutaneously (I.V. if the patient is in shock or in extremis), until blood sugar level is lower than time before--then 25 units per 90 minutes until blood sugar level is under 450.
350-449	Regular insulin, 35 units every 3 hours, given subcutaneously (I.V. if the patient is in shock or in extremis), until blood sugar level is lower than time before--then 25 units every 4 hours until blood sugar level is under 350.
250-349	Regular insulin, 25 units every 4 hours, given subcutaneously (I.V. if the patient is in shock or in extremis), until the blood sugar is under 250--then check twice a day.

If one does a urine sugar at the same time he draws a blood sugar, when the correlations between blood sugars and urine sugars for the patient concerned are made, one can shift over to using urine sugars to judge insulin dose.

2. If there is acetone in the urine, increase saline administration at rate to obtain output of 200 ml. per hour of urine.

3. If pH is below 7.3, give ampule of NaHCarb (44 mEq) hourly times 4 or until pH is above 7.35. (If the serum osmolality is over 350--do NOT give the NaHCarb until the patient is hydrated to less osmolality).

4. If the patient is in coma and/or a known diabetic and blood sugar level is over 500 for an unexplained reason, start to treat for an unexplained infection (could be in urine, lungs, gallbladder, or central nervous system) with:

   a. Chloramphenicol, 6 gm. I.V.
   b. Methicillin, 8 gm. I.V.
   c. Penicillin, 10 million units I.V.

* The current fad is using lower doses of insulin, but I suggest sticking to the "tried and true".

5. Check K every 4 hours and add KCl by volutrol on a 4-hour basis (to invoke this have urine output of at least 80 ml. per hour).

4-hour Reading	Volutrol injection of 150 ml. saline with K added
3 -- 3.9	100 ml.
4 -- 4.5	50 ml.
4.6 -- 5	25 ml.

6. Get lactic acid and if over 3--give methylene blue, 50 mg. I.V., every 6 hours.

7. If after 6 hours blood sugar is over 400, OR osmolality is over 360, OR sodium is over 165, OR lactic acid is over 3--dialyze. (Some may disagree with this but the patient is in such dire straits that something must be done.)

SYSTEM FOR TREATING DISSEMINATING INTRAVASCULAR COAGULATION

At this time I am disenchanted with heparin in this condition and feel intensive treatment of the underlying disease is the only effective therapy. However, if one does use heparin, I suggest using 5000 units dissolved in 500 ml. of saline by slow drip, titrated at a rate that appears to slow oozing from the gums or venopuncture sites. Always test for circulating anticoagulants in what appears to be intravascular clotting as they can be present as well.

If the patient's blood prevents other blood from clotting, use protamine, I. V., alternatively with heparin, based on the desperate philosophy that paradoxical conditions might need paradoxical treatment.

ELECTROCARDIOGRAM

There are so many excellent tests regarding EKG that I feel that a section on EKG reading is unnecessary in this Manual. However, the daily changes that occur should be noted by the responsible physician and with a check (x) on the Critical Care Flowsheet should be described--either on the Progress Notes or specifically brought to this physician's attention.

The extent to which a particular Critical Care Unit wants to go in regard to CONTINGENCY ORDERS for EKG will vary greatly and will have to be decided on an individual Unit basis.

DIAGNOSTIC CONTINGENCY ORDERS FOR ELECTROCARDIOGRAMS:

1. Rhythm change: Draw K and digoxin levels and follow Digoxin Contingency orders (page 196).

2. Digitalis toxicity: Draw K and STOP digitalis preparations. Give K, 40 mEq/liter until K level is at 4.5 and use dilantin, 250 mg. I.V. STAT and then every 6 hours for superventricular arrhythmia.

3. Coronary insufficiency: i.e., evidence of lack of blood to myocardium--bed rest, CPK with isoenzymes every 6 hours times three, SGOT, morphine gr. 1/6, atropine 1/100 for severe chest pain, and monitor O_2 at 6 liters/minute.

4. Coronary occlusion, acute: Order serial EKG, start oxygen 6 liter/minute, morphine, gr. 1/6, atropine 1/100 every 4 hours, CPK with isoenzymes every 6 hours, SGOT daily times two, and use lidocaine as agreed upon by your unit.

5. Auricular fibrillation: If this is a new finding seek specific order from responsible physician as to how to react, i.e., electric shock or digitalis? Usually digitalize and then shock.

6. Flutter: If this is a new finding seek specific orders from the responsible physician as to how to react, i.e., quinidine, pronestyl, or digitalis?

7. Pulmonary embolus (suggestive of): Get chest x-ray, lung scan, LDH with isoenzymes, O_2 at 6 liters/minute, atropine gr. 1/100 if acute chest pain.

8. Other readings: Get proper reaction from attending physician.

9. Multiple premature ventricular contractions (PVC): If over 6/minute give bolus of lidocaine, 50-100 mg., and then run drip of lidocaine, 1-4 mg/min.

10. Sinus tachycardia:
    a. Press on carotid sinus on one side to help establish the diagnosis since this causes rate to slow if the diagnosis is correct.

    b. Propranolol (inderal) 10 mg. by mouth every 6 hours if patient has symptoms and there is no underlying difficulty that will cause lowered cardiac output.

11. Paroxysmal atrial tachycardia:

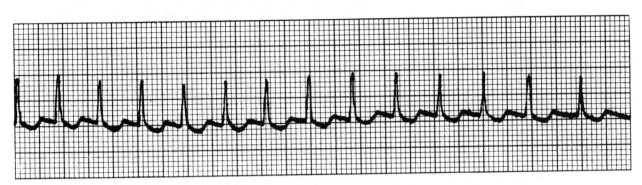

    a. Try Valsalva effort and carotid pressure first -- this will often stop the attack.
    b. Try edrophonium (tensilon) 10 mg. I.V. and then --
    c. Try cedilanid, 4 cc. I.V. and then --
    d. Follow this with oral use of pronestyl, 0.5 gm. by mouth every 6 hours.
    e. Follow this with lidocaine, 500 mg. bolus, then slow drip.
    f. Then consider electrical conversion.

12. Paroxysmal atrial tachycardia with block:

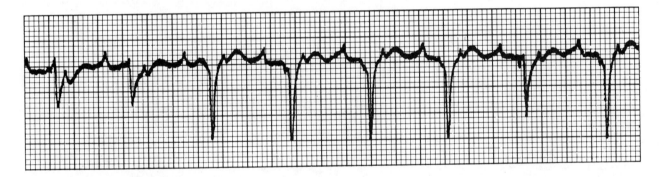

    a. Get digitalis level.
    b. Normalize K.
    c. Give dilantin, 100 mg. I.V. (be sure not to get outside the vein) and repeat every 4 hours times 3. Monitor dilantin levels which should be between 2 and 10.
    d. If the block causes a ventricular rate under 50--use temporary transvenous pacing.

13. Multifocal atrial tachycardia:

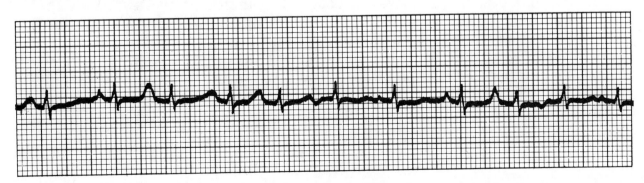

a. Get digoxin level.
b. Normalize K.
c. If **NOT** on digitalis, give cedilanid, 4 cc.
d. If not in heart failure, try propranolol, quinidine, or pronestyl.
e. Do **NOT** use electrical conversion.

14. Atrial flutter:

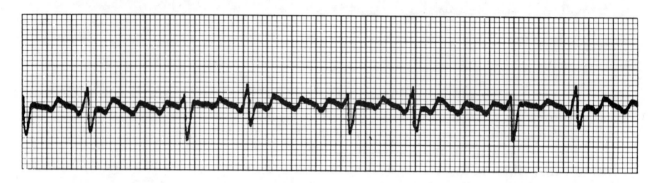

a. Convert with 25 to 100 Watt seconds of direct current shock and follow with quinidine, gr. III, every 6 hours.
b. After conversion, digitalize the patient.
c. Try to maintain conversion by manipulating quinidine, pronestyl, digoxin, and propranolol (inderol).

15. Atrial fibrillation:

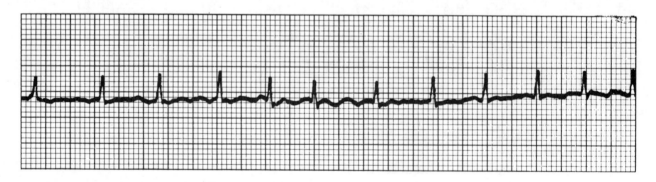

a. Order thyroid studies.
b. Try cardioversion if: No evidence of heart disease.
   Recent mitral valve replacement.
   After treatment for thyrotoxicosis if fibrillation continues
c. If you decide not to convert electrically, digitalize to slow rate to below 100 and they try to convert with quinidine, gr. III every 3 hours for 6 doses and then given on basis to achieve level of 5 to 10 --
d. Digitalize and try procainamide, 0.5 gm. by mouth 4 times a day in patients who cannot tolerate quinidine. You then might try to convert electrically.

16. Ventricular tachycardia:

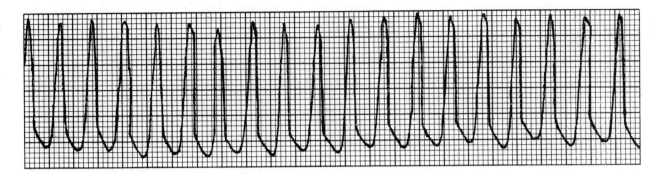

   a. Lidocaine, 100 mg. by bolus, continued by drip at 3-7 mg. per minute. If this does not restore normal rhythm and control premature ventricular contractions --
   b. Give 200 to 400 Watt seconds of current.
   c. If the bursts of ventricular tachycardia are occurring during heart rates under 50, give atropine, one mg. every hour or two.
   d. If this does not make rate more rapid, institute transvenous pacing.
   e. Continue procaine drip, 50 to 250 mg. an hour, for 24 hours after ventricular tachycardia stops and then maintain on pronestyl or quinidine.
   f. If over 250 mgm lidocaine/hour - check levels q 4 hours.

17. Ventricular fibrillation:

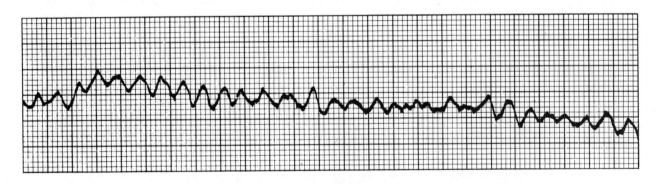

   a. Defibrillate with 400 mg. of Watt seconds of current--given every few minutes until you change the rhythm.
   b. Do external cardiac massage unless there is definitely a good blood pressure (rate).
   c. If the rhythms followed a bradycardia, start transvenous pacing.
   d. Maintain on lidocaine drip and then on oral pronestyl or quinidine.
   e. Maintain circulation with cardiogenic shock system (page 179).

18. Sinus brachycardia: Heart rate under 60 with normal appearing EKG.
   a. Draw a digoxin level and react to it (page 196).
   b. Try atropine, 0.5 to one mg., every 4 hours subcutaneously or I.V.
   c. If more than temporary and patient is having any fainting spells or symptoms--a permanent pacemaker will be necessary. This is often called "sick sinus syndrome".

19. Sinoatrial block:

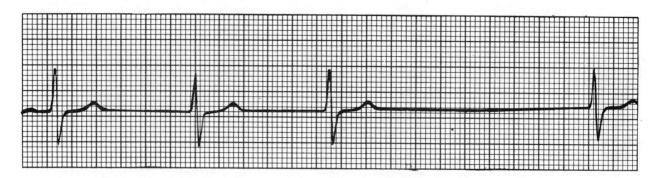

   a. No treatment if only an occasional p wave drops out.

   b. Get digitalis and quinidine levels (quinidine level should be under 10) and treat accordingly if digoxin level is elevated.

   c. If seemingly temporary and associated with other disease--give atropine, 0.5 to 1.0 mg., every 4 hours.

   d. If this does not work, start isuprel, 3 mg. in 300 ml. saline at microdrip rate to increase rate above 60.

   e. If this does not do the trick, start with temporary pacing and you may have to have a permanent pacer placed.

20. First degree block (P-R interval beyond .2 sec.):

   a. Usually not necessary to treat.

   b. Get ASO titer and C-negative protein in young patients as this often occurs with acute rheumatic fever.

21. Second degree block. Mobitz type I (or Wenckebach): Sequential lengthening of P-R interval until ventricular beat drops off.

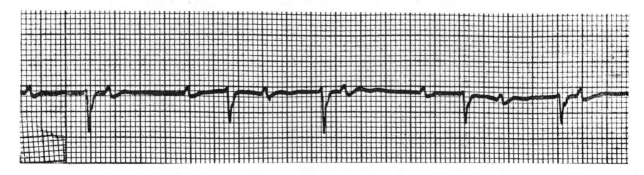

Mobitz type I (Wenckebach) second-degree AV block.

   a. Get digoxin and quinidine levels and discontinue if they are elevated.

   b. May use atropine, 0.5 to 1.0 mg., subcutaneously or I.V. if ventricular rate under 60.

   c. Usually improves as general condition improves.

22. Mobitz type II: heart block without preceding lengthening of the P-R interval.

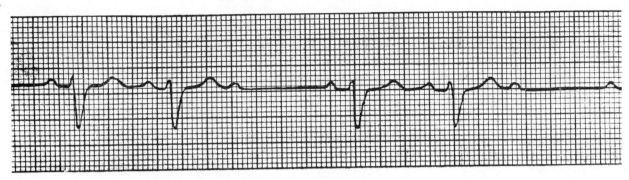

Mobitz type II second-degree AV block.

    a. Unless this is extremely transient and responds to atropine, 0.5 to 1.0 mg. this is an indication for transvenous pacing and probable need for a permanent pacemaker.

23. Third Degree Heart Block: Complete heart block.
    a. No p waves (atrial contractions) are transmitted through to the ventricle.
    b. If there are any symptoms, even in a young patient, this is a prime indication for a permanent transvenous pacemaker.

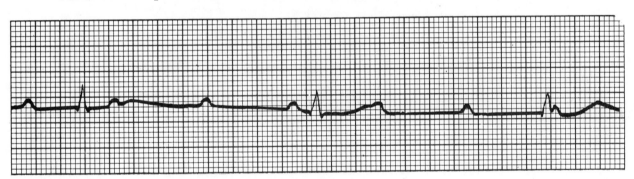

POSSIBLE INDICATIONS FOR ELECTRICAL PACING

1. Paroxysmal atrial tachycardia with block if the block causes a rate under 55 --usually temporary.

2. Sinus bradycardia (usually after coronary) that has resulted in paroxysmal ventricular tachycardia.

3. Bradycardia after conversion of ventricular fibrillation.

4. Symptoms causing sinus bradycardia.

5. Sinoatrial block that is persistent.

6. Second degree heart block (Mobitz type I Wenckebach) that does not respond to treatment.

7. Mobitz type II heart block almost always will need a pacer.

8. Third degree heart block.

POSSIBLE INDICATIONS FOR USE OF ELECTRICAL CONVERSION

START WITH 400 MILLISECONDS--REPEAT AND THEN INCREASE DOSE

1. Paroxysmal atrial tachycardia that has not responded to other measures.

2. Atrial flutter (usually done early).

3. Atrial fibrillation--no evidence of heart disease after treatment for thyrotoxicosis after open heart surgery.

4. Ventricular tachycardia--if bolus of lidocaine not effective.

5. Ventricular fibrillation.

6. Ventricular asystole.

7. Ventricular bradycardia.

NOTES

BACKGROUND ESSAYS

CONTENTS

1. Computerization of this Manual.

2. Essentials of a Critical Care Unit: What--<u>NOT</u> Who or Where.

3. Toward a mission-oriented medical record system.

4. The Rabelaisian school of treating severe infection -- a hopeful paradigm.

5. Simultaneous multiple organ support.

COMPUTERIZATION OF THIS MANUAL

My concepts regarding computers and systems have changed quite a bit since I have been developing and using the Manual, and I no longer think systems and computers are mutually dependent. In other words, one can practice systems as well, and perhaps better, using humans rather than computers. An intelligent, well-paid, aggressive individual on a ward who goes after the laboratory data like a bird dog and who keeps up the flowsheets diligently is probably cheaper, and can do a job helping a physician take care of a patient better than any computer yet devised (with the help of a manual such as this, of course). Therefore I believe that computerization of a Critical Care area can await the development of a "total information system" in a hospital and that for individual tasks modular computers of small cost can usually do the job. Certainly on a priority basis a Unit ought to have plenty of pulmonary artery catheters, cardiac output computers, dialysis machines, aortic pumps, membrane lungs, resin columns, respirators, hyperbaric chambers, and instant laboratory support before they use scarce dollars to buy a fancy computer.

How a manual such as this will fit into a "total information system" of a hospital eventually is detailed in the chapter on the Mission-Oriented Record System (page 226).

For those who do want to computerize the Manual, the initial steps are very simple:

1. Rent time on a time-sharing computer with a terminal that will fit into a telephone on the ward.

2. Have the programmer take the Contingency Order Flowsheet and arrange it so that when a laboratory value falls outside the range indicated after its listing on the Flowsheet a printout of the appropriate page in the Manual is produced by the terminal on the ward.

3. At the end of each shift have the ward secretary punch in the laboratory data for each patient, and the appropriate pages will appear at the telephone terminal.

4. This information can be used for quality control in that the ward secretary can then check the suggested order from the terminal with the written orders on the chart to see how well the Unit is meeting its predetermined system, and, if requested, she can notify the physician of the omissions, or, if authorized, can institute them. After a year's trial of a pilot project of this type, you will be able to move into a phase two type of pilot project and will begin to determine what kind of computerization you might eventually want to invest in.

ESSENTIALS OF A CRITICAL CARE UNIT:

What -- Not Who or Where

During the course of the past 25 years I have had the opportunity to treat patients in ten Critical Care Units located in hospitals in the Milwaukee area. On careful consideration of this experience my conclusion is that there are five essential elements for moderately adequate Critical Care. A hospital Care Committee can work out numerous methods to provide these elements and if they are successful in doing so they will be able to deliver the care a critically ill patient needs, whether he is suffering from gram-negative shock, severe burn, trauma, pulmonary failure, acute renal failure, poisoning, or cardiogenic shock. Above all the Unit must have a clearly delineated system by which these five elements are brought together and made operative. This manual can form the basis of this system.

THE FIVE ESSENTIAL ELEMENTS OF CRITICAL CARE

ONE: The presence at the bedside at all times of someone who knows the patient and his illness intimately.

The effectiveness of this part of a Critical Care System is the ease in spot checking at regular intervals by having a knowledgable person approach the bedside and ask five questions of the responsible person. 1) What is the patient's main problem? 2) What is the patient's underlying disease? 3) What are the results of the last blood gases? 4) What medications are being given? And 5) what is the weight, BUN, Na, K, Hemoglobin, CVP, or pulmonary artery pressure? If these questions can be answered without hesitation--the staffing is adequate. Of course, this entire manual, and particularly the flowsheets, are designed to make this possible.

TWO: There must be a single responsible physician who is in actual, NOT NOMINAL, charge of the patient.

I believe patients in Critical Care areas deserve a physician who has finished his training as the decision maker in critical illness. Whenever residents, interns, or students man a Critical Care Unit, one has to ask himself who is, in fact, making the decisions. If the Teaching Service is set up so that the Professor is actually doing this--fine. If the reality is that he is NOT, is this fair to the patient, and does the patient know he is being treated by an intern, resident, or even a "student"?

A single responsible physician in charge of all the patients in a Critical Care Unit can hardly be the best solution for these patients. It seems to me that it is more logical to have the patient's primary specialist in charge, with mandatory consultations when various organ support systems are used. For instance, while I believe the general surgeon whose patient has ruptured a diverticulum should be able to order the utilization of an artificial kidney and/or a respirator, I also believe in that case the patient will benefit from consultation with the physician trained in respirators and artificial kidneys. Similarly, the open heart surgeon should remain in charge of his postoperative revascularization patients, but if and when serious arrhythmia or pulmonary problems develop the patient should be seen by the original referring cardiologist or internist.

To have an anesthesiologist or internist trained in respirators become the primary physician in charge of all the sick patients in the Critical Care Unit seems illogical, and in hospitals where this happens actual critical care tends to become fragmented because of the natural reluctance of specialists, be they surgeons, cardiologists, cancer chemotherapists, internists, renologists, or primary care specialists to lose control of their patients' destinies.

There has to be an administrative head, of course, but I wonder if he even has to be a physician? With the implementation of a system such as is outlined in this manual, a hospital Staff and Administration should feel secure that its patients are receiving an acceptable standard of care, and by keeping the Critical Care Unit open to all the members of the Staff this standard should be constantly raised from input derived from the various specialties. I am aware that the concept of not having a single person in clinical charge of all patients will run counter to the practice of many excellent Units around the country and, if the single physician can manage it--fine, but the fact remains each patient in a Critical Care Unit should have a primary physician who has finished specialty training as his ultimate decision maker.

THREE: Immediate laboratory backup must be available.

Familiarity with the use of arterial lines and their use in all seriously ill patients is necessary, and the arterial blood they yield must be used to determine blood gases frequently. The same availability must obtain in regard to chest x-rays, electrolyte determinations, and backup regarding arrhythmias that show up on the monitors. Having gotten along fairly well without flow-directed catheters and hemodilution cardiac outputs for many years, I cannot say that at present they are sine qua nons of an adequate Critical Care Unit. However, I have found "happiness is knowing the pulmonary artery pressure, wedge pressure, cardiac output, and peripheral resistance" when one is treating a really seriously ill patient.

FOUR: There must be machine backup.

Here a volume respirator that is available (and for which there is always someone around who can slip in a soft endotracheal tube) is a sine qua non of a Critical Care area. I would hope each Unit in this country is evolving toward hemodialysis, aortic balloon, and hyperbaric oxygen capabilities, but at this point in time a Unit can function without these as long as they have a predetermined plan for hemodialysis, balloon pumping, and hyperbaric oxygen use that can be instituted within several hours by a transfer system, the details of which have been worked out in advance.

FIVE: Critical Care must be given in a humanistic framework.

I have written of this in detail elsewhere* so suffice it to say, in my opinion, anyone who has to die should have the right to die without undue suffering or prolongation and I do not believe a physician ever has to shut off a machine for this to happen.

---

* Waisbren, B.A.: The Function of the Hospital Environment in the Human Endeavor. Arch. Intern. Med. 130: 785-88, 1972.

In addition, the patient should have the right to die in a bed from which he can see the sky, sun, and moon and hear the cars honking outside, and he has every right to have his loved ones at his side, touching him if they wish during the fatal or potentially fatal illness. Isolation cannot be considered good for the health and welfare of a dying patient, and experience with burn patients has demonstrated to us that the family can be in close proximity at all times without its hurting the patient or the delivery of care. The one exception to this may be completely immunodepressed or immunodeficient patients who, however, can be spared visual isolation if they are treated in a plastic life island setup.

Toward a mission-oriented medical record system

BURTON A. WAISBREN, MD

A Mission-Oriented Medical Record System has been found highly practical and useful in the management of hospitalized patients. The MOMRS records are brief and concise without sacrifice of meaningful data. It is designed for a specific mission—to facilitate the management of hospitalized patients and provide for a quality control. The system is compatible for incorporation into a computer program.

The Mission-Oriented Medical Record System (MOMRS) has been designed and developed with *one specific mission* in mind; ie, to facilitate the management of hospitalized patients, especially those in the intensive care units.

The MOMRS was motivated by the pressing need for simplification of the traditional record keeping in view of the growing complexity and volume of laboratory data required in the management of hospitalized patients; also, by the necessity to highlight the important factors in the management of the patient and set up an automatic quality control.

The MOMRS was developed through a series of pilot projects in the Critical Care Unit of the St. Mary's Burn Center in Milwaukee. The system has now been in use for a year, with an experience in over 100 patients.

MOMRS differs from the Problem-Oriented Medical System of Weed[1,2] in that it does not encompass the multiple missions of patient care,

From the Burn Research and Medical Systems, Laboratory, St. Mary's Hospital Burn Center, Milwaukee, Wisconsin.

Presented at the 2nd Annual Meeting of the Society of Critical Care Medicine, May 12, 1973, Pittsburgh, Pa.

medical teaching, and demonstration of thought processes; therefore, it does not require a *detailed* problem-oriented record (data base/problem list/initial plans/progress notes) → medical audit → correction of deficiencies.

The MOMRS record is brief and concise, without sacrifice of meaningful data. It is completely typewritten so it can be read easily and quickly in informing physicians and nurses as to what has happened and what is going on with the patient. The insistence on typewritten records merely recognizes the fact that many physicians have illegible handwriting. MOMRS is compatible for incorporation into a computerized total information system of the hospital and is amenable to an ongoing computerized quality control.

FUNCTIONAL ASPECTS OF MOMRS

The MOMRS required some changes in functions and activities of the physician, nurse, ward secretary, and other personnel of the hospital.[3,4]

The Physician in the MOMRS

The primary functions of a physician do not change in the MOMRS except that he is relieved of considerable writing and record keeping and has more time to practice medicine and supervise other members of the medical team.

The admitting physician, by whatever method he has been trained, does a complete history and physical examination of the patient, dictates the Problems/Data/Solutions for immediate transcription by a ward communicator, and determines the type of Flow Chart to be used. He periodically checks the record, examines the patient, and makes the necessary changes in orders.

Reprinted with permission from: Critical Care Medicine, Vol. 1 No. 5, September-October, 1973, pp. 261-266.

```
                        PROBLEM LIST

        28-year-old white male—Social Security Number 123-45-6789

                                                   Hypothetical
  Date Recorded    Date Solved      Problems       Code Number

     7/11/72                    Acute lobar pneumonia      000716
     7/11/72                    Chronic alcoholism         000213
     7/11/72                    Strong family history      000617
                                   of diabetes
     7/11/72                    Allergic to penicillin     000218
```

Fig. 1—An example of a Problem Sheet (a 28-year-old male with pneumonia).

A new physician may want to use the detailed Problem-Oriented Record System to arrive at the Problems/Data/Solutions of the MOMRS. This is all well and good, but he should do this on separate sheets of paper and summarize his results for the MOMRS. The busy, experienced physician accomplishes the same analysis in his thought processes with certain short cuts developed over years of practice.

The Nurse in the MOMRS

The main change of function for the nurse in the MOMRS is the deletion of all clerical duties and a greater involvement in the management of the patient.[5] Describing the more sophisticated functions of the critical care nurse is outside the scope of this paper. Her function in MOMRS is to review periodically the patient's record, check off the Cardex Order Sheet, and dictate Progress Notes.

The Ward Communicator in the MOMRS

The most significant change in function incorporated in the MOMRS is the assignment of all aspects of record keeping to ward communicators (formerly, ward secretaries and ward clerks). They in fact become an important member of the medical team. An intelligent, aggressive ward communicator must be assigned to each shift. The duties of a ward communicator are: 1) type up the various sections of the MOMRS from the original dictation of the admitting physician, 2) be aware of the overall picture in the management of the patient, 3) fill out all requisitions, 4)

Table 1: Data for inclusion in the Flow Sheet for critical care as compared with coronary care.

CRITICAL CARE

INTAKE (liters)	Blood Pressure	B U N	W B C
OUTPUT (liters)	C. V. P.	Creatinine Clearance	% Stabs
Pao_2	Blood Volume	Serum Osmolality	Culture: Urine E=E. Coli
$Paco_2$	Hematocrit	Urine Osmolality	Blood P=Proteus
pH	Hemoglobin	Na	K=Kleb-Aero.
Lactic Acid	Reticulocyte Count	K	Wound Ps=Pseudo.
$Cao_2 - C\bar{v}o_2$	Platelet Count	Ca	S=Staph.
Tidal Volume	Fibrinogen	F. B. S.	Peak Temperature
pO_2 after 100% O_2	Prothrombin Time	Serum Cortisol	

CORONARY CARE

ECG change	Wedge Pressure
Chest x-ray change	C. V. P.
SGPT	Extra beats
CPK	Prothrombin time (sec.)
LDH	Coumadin
Cardiac Output	

monitor and seek out all the necessary data for the records, 5) keep the record legible in all respects and completely up-to-date.

Ward communicators are trained on the job by the nurses and physicians, as well as by other experienced ward communicators. The nurses and physicians on the ward constantly refer to the records of their patients, and in their scrutiny verify the accuracy of the ward communicator. In the process, the ward communicator receives in-service training.

One of the pleasures of the MOMRS for the physician making rounds is to arrive on the ward and be greeted by a communicator who is worried about a low serum potassium. Encouragement of this type of involvement has proven to be the stimulus to the development of trained, active, useful ward communicators.

In our experience one ward communicator can maintain the records of ten patients. During the day shift when there is the most activity she should be helped by a ward communicator trainee. The amount of help required depends on the organizational structure record keeping of the hospital.

As inevitable computerization takes place, the job of a ward communicator will constantly change and the flexibility to act successfully as the human interface between various computerized programs as they develop, will be the *sine qua non* of the position.

DESCRIPTION OF MOMRS

The MOMRS is divided into four sections: 1) Problem Sheet, 2) Flow Sheets (individualized for various diseases and conditions), 3) Cardex Order Sheet, and 4) Progress Notes.

Section 1—Problem Sheet

The problems as dictated by the examining physician are listed on the cover or top sheet of the records (Problem Sheet) by a ward communicator. Problems are listed in the order of importance, with space for the date recorded, date solved, and the hypothetical code number for each problem (*Fig. 1*). This Problem Sheet is kept up-to-date by the ward communicators, as they periodically check the Progress Notes and the Flow Sheet to see if any of the problems have been resolved or if new problems have arisen, and make the proper notations.

Section 2—Flow Sheets

In the management of an individual patient, there are certain pertinent data which should be followed on a day-to-day basis or at more frequent intervals. In the MOMRS this data is kept on a Flow Sheet, with abnormal values circled. A typical Flow Sheet for a patient with pneumo-

Fig. 2—An example of a Flow Sheet (for the same patient as in Figure 1).

THE FLOW SHEET

Name—JOHN DOE		Admitted—7/11/72		Diagnosis—PNEUMONIA	
HOSPITAL DAY	1	2	3	4	5
Maximum temp.	100° F.	100° F.			
Sputum culture	Pneumo.	neg.			
Blood culture	Pseudo +	neg.			
X-ray changes	Infiltrate	no change			
EKG	Normal	—			
WBC	18,000	14,000			
% polys	90%	65%			
% monocytes	—	4%			
% eosinophiles	—	—			

Other data to be put in by clinician—these can be added as the case develops.

Serum bilirubin	+1.0		3.2		
BSP	22%				
SGPT	88		30		
LDH	60		40		
Drug tolerance	O.K.	O.K.	O.K.		
Sensorium	clear	D.T.s	D.T.s		

CARDEX ORDER SHEET

Date	Activating Initials (Optional)	Orders	Dose	Frequency Daily	(DAILY OVERLAYS) Shift 1	2	3
7/11/72		Erythromycin	0.5 gm. P.O.	q.i.d.	X	X	X
		Elixir of terpin hydrate	1 tsp. P.O.	t.i.d.	X	X	X
		Librium	10 mg. P.O.	t.i.d.	X	X	X
		Daily C.B.C.			X		
		Sputum culture	STAT && q.o.d.		X		
		Chest x-ray	7/11-7/14-7/23		X		
		EKG			X		
		BSP			X		
		Chloral hydrate	gr. 7½ H.S.p.r.n.				X
7/12/72		Serum bilirubin	1 min. & total		X		
7/12/72		May restrain if necessary					

Fig. 3—An example of a Cardex Order Sheet (for the same patient as in Figures 1 and 2).

nia is illustrated in Figure 2. It is the responsibility of the ward communicator to make the proper entries as the data becomes available. Inasmuch as the same type of data is not applicable to every patient, the Flow Sheet must be tailor-made to include the pertinent data relative to the specific condition or disease being treated. The same Flow Sheet cannot be used for myocardial infarction, diabetic coma, bleeding ulcer, renal failure, shock, and a critically ill patient with multiple injuries and multiple organ failure. The variables in data are illustrated in Table 1. In the MOMRS the Medical Staff decides on the Flow Sheets necessary to cover particular situations. Physician Committees, with expertise in specific conditions or diseases, are delegated the responsibility of setting up appropriate Flow Sheets.

The MOMRS Flow Sheet is designed to reflect only highly pertinent data. Therefore, in the planning and development of MOMRS there is the problem as to what to do with the vast amount of information gathered on each patient, which has been part of the traditional medical record. This data cannot clutter up the MOMRS and should be kept at its point of origin for retrieval if needed. In our experience, it takes physicians and nurses a while to get used to not seeing every-

thing in the record of the patient. Therefore, during the transitional period to the MOMRS, a traditional record can be kept simultaneously, or the laboratory reports can be kept on file on the ward. When the staff and the attending physician gradually realize that they do not need all of the data, they will consent to leaving unessential data in the laboratory files.

Section 3—Cardex Order Sheet

The Cardex Order Sheet *(Fig. 3),* itemizes all medication, laboratory procedures, and other orders for the patient as typed by a ward communicator from the dictated orders of the admitting physician. This sheet contains an overlay for the nurse on each shift to check or initial when each order is executed. These checks or initials are the only writing the nurse does in the MOMRS. At the end of each shift, the ward communicators verify that all orders have been checked or initialed. All new orders are entered on the Cardex Order Sheet as they are dictated. The Cardex Order Sheet must be kept highly legible at all times and are re-typed as often as necessary. Each day, the check-off overlay is renewed. Used sheets and overlays are put to the back of the record for future reference if needed.

PROGRESS NOTES

7/11/72	28-year-old white male—Social Security Number 123-45-6789

PROBLEMS: Acute lobar pneumonia
Chronic alcoholism
Strong family history of diabetes
Allergic to penicillin

DATA: Fever 104° F.
Rusty sputum
Consolidation left lower lobe by x-ray
and physical findings
Blood pressure 160/80
Pulse 100
Heart normal

SOLUTIONS: Blood culture
Sputum culture and Gram smear
Erythromycin 0.5 gm. P.D. q.i.d. × 4
Bed rest with bathroom privileges
Regular diet
Pneumonia flow sheet
SMA with electrolyte
Daily F.B.S.

Armin Burton, M.D.
Admitting Physician

7/12/72 X-ray report—consolidation of left lower lobe/John James,
Radiologist.

7/12/72 EKG report—normal EKG/Sam Sneed, Cardiology.

7/12/72 Gram smear of sputum—typical of Pneumococcus/Jane Doe,
Lab. Tech.

7/12/72 Fever has broken—10 P.M.—patient much improved since
admission/Alice Bahr, Nurse.

7/13/72 Classic response to classic pneumonia but patient seems to
be developing the D.T.s. If he gets too active he
may be restrained.

Armin Burton, M.D.

Fig. 4—An example of Progress Notes (for the same patient as in Figures 1, 2 and 3).

The format of the Cardex Order Sheet serves as a quality control in management.

Section 4—Progress Notes

The Progress Notes of MOMRS *(Fig. 4)* contain the Problems/Data/Solutions as originally dictated by the admitting physicons with notes of important developments during the course of hospitalization. A physician, nurse, laboratory technician, physiotherapist, social worker; whoever has pertinent information as to the progress of the patient dictates an entry to the Progress Notes. Every entry is related to a listed problem. Every entry is brief and to the point. Anyone connected with the management of the patient can at a glance, within a second or two, see what is happening to the patient.

The physician in charge of the patient on his daily rounds can look at the Problem List, the Flow Sheet, the Cardex Order Sheet; talk to and examine the patient; refer to the Progress Notes; and then dictate his clinical impression. At such time, he may consider one of the problems solved, or he may issue a new order or two.

Problem	Code No. Assigned
Acute lobar pneumonia	= 1
Chronic alcoholism	= 2
Family history of diabetes	= 3
Penicillin allergy	= 4
Data	
Gram-positive lancet-shaped Diplococci	= 1
Initial temperature—102° F.	= 2
Infiltration of right upper lobe x-ray	= 3
Solutions	
Erythromycin—0.5 gm. P.O. q.i.d.	= 1
Librium—10 mg. P.O. t.i.d.	= 2
Chest x-ray × 3	= 3
Elixir of terpin hydrate—1 tsp. P.O. t.i.d.	= 4

Fig. 5—An example of how the MOMRS can be computerized. Problems, data, and solution are assigned code numbers (as above). With these numbers and descriptions the programmer can easily program any of many computers so that, when a ward communicator types in—PROBLEMS: 1, 2, 3, 4; DATA: 1, 2, 3; SOLUTIONS: 1, 2, 3, 4—these numbers can be stored under the Social Security number of the patient, on a disk or tape. When the patient is readmitted, a request for past medical history and hospitalization, made via teletype from any terminal connected to the computer, would receive this reading: Soc. Sec. No. 123-45-6789; name—John Doe; admitted St. Mary's Hospital 7/11/72 with lobar pneumonia; chronic alcoholism; family history of diabetes; penicillin allergy; positive Gram Stain for lancet-shaped Diplococci; initial temperature 102° F.; 7/11/72 x-ray—infiltration right upper lobe; 7/21/72—x-ray cleared; treated with erythromycin, librium, elixir terpin hydrate; total laboratory results available on further request.

COMPUTERIZATION

The MOMRS is designed for immediate use and storage in a traditional medical record room, with possible adaptation to the medical record room of the future with all records stored on disks or magnetic tape.[6] In the medical record room of the future, selective printout of past events could be made when a patient is readmitted to the hospital. Details of such computerization are outside the scope of this paper, but suffice it to say that the Problems/Data/Solutions of each patient can all have designated code numbers, and concomitant with keeping the chart current, the ward communicators can place numbers on tape or a disk that will be available either for recall, to act as "requisitions", or to go into a quality control computer (Fig. 5). The MOMRS charts will serve as a data bank for the computerization step, both for the total information system and for an on-going quality control.

Any computer facility that offers time sharing will have a large enough computer to do an initial pilot project with this record system. These will be in the range of the IBM 360 series. All large cities have companies or schools with these capabilities. The phase II or actual total computerization of a record room in conjunction with a total information system of the hospital will be a more complicated problem.

SUMMARY

The MOMRS has been found highly practical and useful in the management of hospitalized patients at the St. Mary's Burn Center. It has improved the quality of medical care by constantly relating treatment to diagnosis. MOMRS has not only reduced the amount of data required in the medical record of a patient, but has relieved the physician and nurse of all record-keeping duties. The ward communicators assume all record-keeping responsibilities.

REFERENCES

1. Weed LL: Medical Records, Medical Education, and Patient Care, Cleveland, Press of Case Western Reserve University, 1969.
2. Hurst JW, Walker HK: The Problem-Oriented System, New York, MEDCOM, Inc., 1972.
3. Waisbren BA: Designing a modern hospital: a physician's point of view. Delaware Med J 43:102-107, 1971.
4. Waisbren BA: Care of the critically ill: the systems method. Hosp Med Staff 1: Feb., 1972.
5. Waisbren BA: The function of the hospital environment in the human endeavor. Arch Intern Med 130:785-788, 1972.
6. Waisbren BA: Towards a systematized, computerized outpatient department. (submitted for publication.)

THE RABELAISIAN SCHOOL OF TREATING SEVERE INFECTION
-- A HOPEFUL PARADIGM *

"Thou doeth what thou wilt."

-Francois Rabelais (1490-1553)

It seems appropriate to start a discussion regarding the art of treating patients with serious infections with some attention to defining "art" as we shall use it. Webster's Unabridged Dictionary defines art as follows: "Art is the systematic application of knowledge or skill in affecting a desired result"[3]. From here we might turn to John Stuart Mill, founder of Utilitarianism, who said, "Art in general consists of the truth of science arranged in the most convenient order for practice, instead of the order which is most convenient for thought"[4]. Tolstoy puts it more simply, "Art is an activity that produces beauty"[5]. This definition would seem to suffice for our purpose as long as we can define beauty. Edmund Burke gives us help here with his remark that "Beauty is something that gives a sense of joy in beholding"[6]. Shakespeare adds a remark which emphasizes that art must be amenable to proof when he says in his 11th Sonnet, "O, how much more doth beauty beauteous seem, by that sweet ornament which truth doth give"[7]. In these contexts we can define the art of treating patients as a systematic application of knowledge in order to give one the joy of beholding a truly well patient and, as we shall discuss, the patient must be well in more contexts than merely being free of invading bacteria. Finally, in defining art we must not forget comment about the artist. Yehudi Menuhin[8] emphasized that the great artist "allows his inspiration a certain free rein which, emerging from his supreme discipline, is a reminder of a human abandon, impulse, and surrender".

Now let us turn to the man after whom we name the system of treatment we are going to describe. Rabelais was first and foremost a physician. He lived in the 16th century (1490-1553). His skill as a physician probably allowed him the freedom to be an individualist and to write his classic, almost heretical, works because of the fact that he always was the personal physician of those who could protect him[9]. We named our system after Rabelais because of his humanism, good humor, the enthusiastic approach to life of his two main characters, Gargantua, the winsome giant, and Pantagruel the clown, and, perhaps, because the system might require the return to the medical battlefield of only a slightly modified Renaissance man[10].

A school of art must have a series of principles upon which it is based and the Rabelaisian school of therapy of severe infections is no exception.

The first principle is called the "tempo" principle. It states that upon initial contact with the patient the physician makes a careful determination in his own mind as to how long the patient will live if the present course of the

---

* A paradigm as used in this essay is a system that is unprecedented enough to gain adherents and open-ended enough to leave problems for those adherents to solve [2]

disease goes on unchecked. He then sees to it that everything reasonable that can possibly be done to help the patient is done within that time period. If the patient appears to have only a few hours to live, everything is done at once. If the disease seems to be progressing at a slower rate, different modalities may be added in the order of their reasonableness to afford the physician the luxury of determining how effective each might be. The patients I am going to tell you about in a few moments were all of the allegro type. However, on an overall basis most patients with infections may be moderato or progress largo.

The second principle is the "individual therapist" principle or, put another way, in the Rabelaisian system, the artist does the painting. Just as the actual thrust of the sword at the moment of truth in the bull ring is done by the matador, the moment of truth in the treatment of a severely ill patient arrives when the physician in charge actually writes the orders as to what is to be done. Nothing cools artistic ardor more swiftly than the remark by an intern, student, or resident when he is being told to write an order, ". . but if this is such a good treatment why haven't I read about it in the New England Journal of Medicine?" The trainees among the audience will be muttering at this last remark, "But how can I learn if I do not have actual control of the patient?" My answer is very simple, "John Stephans of Calcar (the artist who did the original paintings for Vesalius) and El Greco were both students of Rubens and went on to great things on their own, but we all know that they did not paint the main parts of Rubens' pictures".

The third principle is "treat the Gestalt"[11]. To achieve this the artist must bring in his entire entourage of apprentices and associates. While Rubens always did the faces his apprentices painted in many of the details and embellished his broad outlines. To treat the Gestalt of an infection the full range of laboratory, social welfare, nursing, and trainees must be incorporated in an overwhelming effort. In this context some words must be said about the isolation of the patient. It is ironic that many of our highly scientific Medical Centers that demand a P-value of .001 before a medication is given, have accepted carte blanche the concept that most patients with severe illness-not only those with severe infections--must be isolated from their families and friends. The burden of proof that such isolation helps the patient or that its being ignored is harmful is certainly on its proponents, because I am sure all of us would agree that isolation in a hospital often means isolation from good care and from the one modality that many patients deserve more than anything else--that is, to die in the company of people who love them. Nowhere does this seems more true than in the field of burns, in which the many Centers which have spent literally thousands of dollars to create practically sterile environments have failed to show that this tremendous effort has produced better results than those achieved in the few Burn Centers where patients' families and friends are allowed to support each other during the entire grueling experience. [12, 13]

While concentrating on the external Gestalt we also must not forget the milieu interieur originally emphasized by Claude Bernard[1]. Keeping the blood volume, the electrolyte balance, the cardiac output, the clotting mechanisms, the body defenses, and the endocrine balance normal are as much a part of the art of treating patients with severe infections as are the attention paid to prescribing antibiotics[14]. By the same token constant monitoring of all these parameters is as necessary as daily cultures, so that the physician always know what the true Gestalt is. Thus the physician has to communicate with the patient and family, as well as with his staff and laboratory in order to meet the Gestalt treatment aspect of the Rabelaisian method.

The fourth principle is called the "Gargantuan" principle after the giant created by Rabelais [10]. It states that a seriously ill patient should be treated with the maximum tolerated dosages of multiple agents [15]. The field of infectious diseases has been burdened too long by Ehrlich's fallacious dream, which assumes that because most infections are caused by a single pathogen that they may be cured by a magic bullet that attacks this pathogen [16]. Many observations give the lie to this dream. The most obvious ones are that, while virulent microorganisms such as Meningococci, Pneumococci, and the tubercle bacillus are ubiquitious in our society, on a relative basis the combinations of circumstances that allow them to cause disease are rare. The few situations such as "garden variety" pneumococcal pneumonia, in which a magic bullet such as penicillin works, can no longer be called severe infections, so they are outside the scope of this presentation. The Gargantuan principle should be applied not only to dosage where it is reasonable to expect the highest tolerated dose to have the best chance to reach relatively inaccessible bacteria, but the principle also should be applied by using multiple agents, which will be able to attack the invading bacteria at various susceptible metabolic sites [16,17,18]. Here might be the place to try to lay to rest that old saw that multiple antibiotics should not be used because they inhibit each other. Undoubtedly, chloramphenicol in vitro will decrease the killing rate of penicillin on Enterococci but at the same time the penicillin is potentiating the inhibitory rate of the chloramphenicol [18,19,20]. Whether killing rapidly or inhibiting at a lower dose is more important in a specific infection remains most because conflicting clinical studies can be found in the literature [19,21]. Furthermore, when a patient such as I am going to tell you about is seen, the problem can be solved by adding a third agent such as streptomycin or gentamicin, which will again increase killing [22].

If we accept the thesis that for purposes of penetration the dose at the upper end of the toleration curve should be used, chloramphenicol must be mentioned in particular, because of the campaign of calumny to which it has been subjected. Statistics show that the rate of aplastic anemia with chloramphenicol is approximately the same as the rate of anaphylaxis with penicillin [23]. Yet chloramphenicol has been assaulted on the floor of Congress, as well as by Professors of Medicine who happened to have seen more than their share of aplastic anemia because of their specialties and eminence. It is a tribute to the courage and good sense of the American physician that he has continued to use this drug in high dosage for his seriously ill patients in spite of this unprecedented propaganda campaign [24]. I am sure many of you have had the experience that I have had at least once a month, in which, at the bedside of a dying septic patient and having just ordered among other things, eight grams of chloramphenicol and twenty million units of penicillin. I am asked by the intern, nurse, or chief resident, "But Doctor, aren't you afraid that the patient will get aplastic anemia and that you will be sued?" My answer is always the same, "Yes, I am afraid the patient will get aplastic anemia and that I may be sued, but the patient's condition is such that he can afford to take a one in fifty thousand chance that he will get aplastic anemia in view of the potential good the chloramphenicol may do him and I have had to learn to live with my fear that I might get sued." [23,25].

The fifth principle of the Rabelaisian school is really borrowed from the father of modern pathology, Giovanni Morgagni[26], who, in his De Salibus, published in 1761, pointed out that to understand and treat a disease one must go directly to its seat or center. And of course, Ambroise Pare[27] had shown the way 150 years before when he stated, "Chyrugery is an art, which teacheth the way by reason, how by the operation of the hand, we may cure, prevent, and mitigate disease . . ."

The principle, more simply stated, is that active attack must be made by surgery or other means at the heart of the disease. It has not been a rare occasion for me, and I assume for many of you in the audience, to be called to manage a patient with intra-abdominal sepsis from a ruptured viscus wherein the first order of business has to be immediate surgery to sew up a tear in the bowel. Similarly one of the most gratifying experiences in my memory is observing the almost immediate return of a demonstrable blood pressure in a woman in severe Gram-negative shock when the uterine veins were clamped just prior to the removal of her infected uterus[28]. Thus, this principle always makes the artful therapist ask himself, "Am I treating the cause of the immediate problem as well as the cause of the cause of the immediate problem?"

The sixth principle is that treatment must be given in the framework of a predetermined system. Recent demands made by outside agencies such as the American Hospital Association[29] and the Federal Government[30] make presentation of demands for systems as a suggested principle anachronistic because quality assurance programs, that will themselves demand systems, are being made mandatory in all hospitals. These are to check, in a predetermined manner, how each defined problem is handled. The "predetermined check list" will inevitably become the framework of the systems of treatment that we will use in each hospital. We can only hope that the systems to be used will be developed artfully in the sense of the word as we are discussing it, by the physicians who are going to do the treating; and that each system of treatment will have within it the elements of any good system, i.e., capacity to change as a result of feedback and a broad enough boundary to allow for alternative pathways and for many systems within the "system"[31]. These systems, hopefully, will be undergoing constant refinement, evaluation, and change.

Having presented the six principles of the Rabelaisian school we shall now tell stories that illustrate them. I have been saddened and somewhat amused by the tremendous antianecdotal bias of some of our current medical journals, that seem to take pride in the number of anecdotal papers they reject, while at the same time their scholarly editors are, or should be, devotees of Chaucer, Shakespeare, and the Bible, that are but collections of beautifully expressed anecdotes that have a lot to teach us. Why not use then, medical anecdotes which, as I mentioned in the introduction, are in fact used as medical teaching tools in the corridors and lunch rooms of all our hospitals. I am not proposing that these be the only methods by which we teach, only that they not be cast out of our teaching armamentarium. The four anecdotes are interesting cases seen during the past 3 months and they illustrate systems we use for severe burns and for severe undiagnosed infection in immunodepressed patients.

ANECDOTE 1: The patient was a 26-year-old police ambulance driver who was trapped in a burning ambulance and suffered deep second and third degree burns over 74% of his body. He was admitted to St. Mary's Burn Center in November, 1974, without discernible blood pressure. Resuscitation was accomplished within

24 hours by a multiple organ support system which included, during these first 24 hours, 25 liters of fluid, 180 gm. of salt, hyperbaric oxygen, hemodialysis, balloon aortic pumping and a volume respirator with PEEP through a tracheostomy [32]. A prophylactic system against sepsis was then invoked which included, by daily infusion, 6 gm. of chloramphenicol; 8 gm. of methicillin; 10 million units of penicillin G; polymyxin B, given on the basis of the daily blood urea nitrogen concentration; pooled transfer factor; gamma globulin; and a multivalent whole cell Gram-negative and Candida heat-killed vaccine [32,33,34]. Although under this he achieved a brisk rise in immunoglobulins and T cell percentage, he then developed a septicemia with Serratia marcescens on the sixth hospital day. This was successfully treated with white blood cell infusion; oxytetracycline, 6 gm. per day; and gentamicin, 200 mg. per day, even though he developed a toxic hepatitis, presumably from the intravenous oxytetracycline [35]. By the third week in the hospital he had stabilized somewhat under a program of maximum tolerated dosages of antibiotics, hyperalimentation [36], and intense emotional support by his wife and family, who were at his bedside continuously. The patient was alert during all of this time and enormously cooperative. Chronic lactic acidosis, in spite of all attempts to encourage cellular respiration by methylene blue [37] and vitamin C, indicated his continued precarious state, and he died on the 40th hospital day of overwhelming Escherichia coli septicemia and lactic acidosis.

COMMENT: Was everything possible done to and for this unfortunate young man? Of course not, but it was a reasonable and predetermined method of trying to save a patient who fell in a statistical group that our usual treatment had no chance of saving. He clearly understood and accepted the efforts that were being made.

ANECDOTE 2: The patient was a 48-year-old woman seen at St. Michael's Hospital in Milwaukee in January, 1975. She had developed classic myasthenia gravis three months before and had been hospitalized at another hospital during the first two weeks of December, 1974, during which time a thymoma and a very low blood count had been found [40]. She left that hospital against advice and was admitted to St. Michael's Hospital on December 21st with profound weakness, a temperature of 104° F., a white blood count of 1000, and a left lower lobe pneumonia. In spite of tracheostomy, methicillin, keflin, cleocin, gentamicin, and penicillin G her pneumonia progressed to a lung abscess and her white blood count had fallen to 600, with 20% polymorphonuclear cells found. A bone marrow study suggested a maturation arrest of the white cell series. A specimen obtained by bronchial brush had failed to reveal any pathogenic bacteria or fungi.

The following sequence was suggested and followed: streptomycin, 0.5 gm., intravenously, to treat possible tubercle bacilli; amphotericin B, 25 mg., to treat possible fungi; lincomycin, 6 gm., to treat bacteroides and staphylococcus; gamma globulin, 20 cc.; a concentrated white blood cell infusion; and removal of the spleen and thymoma [41]. This was all accomplished within 24 hours. The patient made an immediate response, both in regard to the myasthenia gravis and white blood count. She was off the respirator in 48 hours. Within a week she had normal muscle strength and a normal white blood count. Her lung abscess responded to therapy with chloramphenicol, which was given when an E. coli suggested itself as the procurable pathogen. The final tragic irony of this story is that the patient suddenly dropped dead as she was about to leave the hospital. We were not able to determine if the cause was a sudden allergic reaction, a pulmonary embolus, or cardiac arrhythmia.

COMMENT: This case is illustrative of the use of the Rabelaisian system before the therapist knew the details of the disease he was treating. Even though we had not been aware of reports of the combination of myasthenia gravis, agranulocytosis, splenomegaly, and thymoma having been reported in the literature before treatment was instituted, following the Morgagni principle of attacking the apparent seat of the disease did seem reasonable, and in this case appeared to be life-saving [40, 41].

ANECDOTE 3: The patient was a 24-year-old man with known granulomatous disease of the adult [42]. He had been treated successfully four years ago for simultaneous lung, liver, and brain abscesses, from which cultures were negative, with a one month's course of the daily infusion of 8 gm. of chloramphenicol; 8 gm. of lincomycin; 120 mg. of gentamicin; 10 cc. of gamma globulin; and 3 liters of modified hyperalimentation. During the ensuing three years he had responded to three similar courses of therapy, given for vicious cellulitis. He had been maintained prophylactically on oral oxacillin, pooled transfer factor, and a whole-cell heat-killed multivalent vaccine, which contained gram-negative bacilli, staphylococci, and candida. He had been actively working as a cement mason. During mid 1974 he became despondent over an unrequited love affair and stopped his regular visits for transfer factor and vaccine.

He was admitted to Mount Sinai Hospital in December, 1974, with a pneumonia which progressed to cause his death in 17 days, in spite of initial daily therapy with polymyxin B, 150 mg.; lincomycin, 4 gm.; chloramphenicol, 4 gm.; and gamma globulin, 10 cc., to which was added as the lack of response was apparent, daily cytosine arabinoside, 175 mg.; streptomycin, one gm.; isoniazid, 100 mg.; keflin, 8 gm.; and amphotericin B, 20 mg. Autopsy revealed a pure aspergillosis pneumonia that had not yielded positive cultures until a fiberoptic bronchoscopy obtained specimen grew a few colonies of this fungus after the sixth hospital day.

COMMENT: Retrospectively, while the life of this vibrant young man was undoubtedly prolonged by the Rabelaisian therapy he received, we ultimately failed him by not providing him with enough emotional support for him to accept the disappointments that appear in the Gestalt of an individual with a chronic disease. Had we done so he might have survived until he could have been given the bone marrow transplant that might have cured his disease [43].

ANECDOTE 4: The patient was a 17-year-old Latino girl who was known to have had lupus erythematosus for two years, during which time her disease had barely been controlled by generous doses of corticosteroids. She was admitted to the Emergency Room of St. Luke's Hospital in November, 1974, with a respiratory arrest, a high fever, and a small area of infiltration of the left base. She was treated by assisted volume respiration, penicillin, cephalosporin, and gentamicin. However, she became progressively worse in spite of supportive care and one gram of Cytoxan, given to her because of a presumptive diagnosis of lupus encephalitis [44].

When seen two weeks after admission she had a temperature of 106º F., a white blood count of 3000, and blood pressure of 100/80. She had a chest tube in which was draining from a bronchopleural fistula, pus which grew Pseudomonas aeruginosa. She remained in deep coma and without any respiratory attempts on her own. Her pupils were widely dilated but they did react to light. She had been maintained on 100 mg. of hydrocortisone per day and was in good electrolyte balance.

The following medications were administered over the next 12 hours: amphotericin B, 20 mg., for possible Candidiasis; cytosine arabinoside, 75 ml., for Herpes encephalitis [45,46]; polymyxin B, 75 mg., and gamma globulin, 10 cc., for Pseudomonas infection [47]; lincomycin, 4 gm., for Staphylococci and Bacteroides; Kafazol, 6 gm., for Enterobacteria [48]; 6 gm. carbenicillin; and a white blood cell infusion to try to normalize phagocytosis until the bone marrow recovered from the Cytoxan. These were all ordered to be administered over a 12-hour period on the basis of the "tempo" principle (vide supra) and because of the desire to prevent central nervous system damage as well as to affect survival. Just as the last of the ordered medications had been infused the patient went into a circulatory collapse, which necessitated a 12-hour course of an isoproterenol drip. Following this she became afebrile and gradually has gotten better until at the time of this writing (two months later) she is off the respirator and seems more alert each day. The referring physician has maintained her on keflin and gentamicin and did not readminister the amphotericin B, polymyxin B, cytosine arabinoside, gamma globulin, or carbenicillin when she came out of shock. The white blood count has returned to normal.

COMMENT: This case illustrates the fact that one has to treat possibilities and that when treatment is done he may not know what he has treated, if his treatment was successful, or whether he did the patient a favor by treating him at all. Being able to live with these uncertainities is one indispensable characteristic of the Rabelaisian therapist. In this case, our guess is that a Herpes encephalitis responded to a fortunately timed dose of cytosine arabinoside but obviously this is only a guess.

Up to now perhaps we have concentrated on art and stories to the partial exclusion of science and the reader will have to determine if these stories gave him as clear a picture of the Rabelaisian system as if it had been presented more didactically. We will now turn to the second part of our title, "A hopeful paradigm", in order to try to bring the Rabelaisian school in under the protective umbrella of science. The word "paradigm" means many things to many people but we are using it as elaborated by Kunn, who defines a paradigm as "a system unique enough to strike a responsive chord among our colleagues and open-ended enough for these colleagues to develop new ideas and methods through its use."[2]. The Rabelaisian system may be defined as a hopeful paradigm because it might strike a chord among physicians whose experience has indicated to them that, in many situations, what actually has to be done for a patient is based on its reasonableness rather than on a rigid "proof of efficacy" of the modality being considered. This proof of efficacy criteria for the use of modalities seems to have developed from interpretations of the writings of a group of 19th century investigators, which included Claude Bernard Pasteur, Erhlich, Helmholtz, and Arthus [1,16,49,50]. These writings have been interpreted to mean that patients should be treated on the basis of rigidly controlled experiments performed on human beings. On the other hand, using reasonableness, hunch, and ever-changing systems as a basis for treatment seems more consistent with the works of 20th century scientists such as Planck[51], Weiner[52], von Bertalanffy[31], Shannon[53], and Kunn[2]. Just as C. P. Snow[54] has called for a meetings of minds between scientists and politicians, perhaps now is the time for a meeting of minds between physicians and these 20th century scientists. In order for the physicians to approach this meeting they will have to learn more about quantum, cybernetics, open-ended systems, and communication feedbacks[31, 51, 52, 53]. They also will have to learn to transform the description of diseases into paradigms that are amenable to multifactorial analysis. For this to happen the patients, their diseases, and their external environment will have to be described with a series of weighted number combinations and indices. Included in these mathematical models will have to be numerous baselines[55, 56] for use to constantly correlate with the ongoing changes in the defined systems that feedback, humanism, and the absence of double-blind studies will demand.

It should be apparent that the Rabelaisian paradigm, that we have only sketchily outlined, is only one among many that may be used as the basis of treatment and severe diseases. There will be some among you who will favor an entirely different approach. I only hope that it can be agreed that each such paradigm has clearly stated principles and that the eventual presentation of data be in a manner amenable to a sophisticated multifactor analysis that will allow us to study patients without experimenting on them.

In summary, I have discussed the art of treating severe infections by presenting the principles of a system or paradigm, named Rabelaisian after the famous Renaissance humanistic physician. This is based on six broad principles which are: the "tempo" principle that states that all possible treatment should be administered before the patient dies; the "individual therapist" principle that states that therapy is in fact administered by a single dedicated individual whose involvement is total; the "Gestalt" principle that states that the patient, as well as his total environment, must be subjected to humanistic management; the "Gargantuan" principle which decrees, within set limits, the highest possible dosages of multiple agents must be used to treat infections in which single agents might not be effective; the "Morgagni - Pare" principle that states the heart of the disease must be actively attacked, by surgery if necessary, and the "systems" principle which expects the entire treatment to be within the framework of a well-defined system that is amenable to multiple factor analysis, feedback, and constant change.

REFERENCES

1. Bernard, Claude: An Introduction to the Study of Experimental Medicine. Trans. H.C. Greene. Macmillan Co., 1927.
2. Kunn, T.S.: The Structure of Scientific Revolution. Univ. of Chicago Press, 1962, p. 10.
3. Webster's Unabridged Dictionary. 2nd Ed. 1955.
4. Mill, John Stuart: Collected Works. Toronto and London, 1963.
5. Tolstoy, L.: What Is Art and Essays on Art. Trans. by World's Classics Series, Oxford University Press, 1930.

240

6. Burke, E.: The Works of the Right Honorable Edmund Burke. Vol. 1. London, 1906.

7. Shakespeare's Eleventh Sonnet.

8. Menuhin, Yehudi: Art as hope for humanity. Saturday Review/World, Dec. 14, 1974.

9. Green, T.M.: Rabelais. A Study in Comic Courage. Prentice-Hall Inc., New Jersey, 1970.

10. Rabelais, Francois: The Histories of Gargantua and Pantagruel. Trans. by J.M. Cohen. Penquin Books, 1963.

11. Koffka, Kurt: Principles of Gestalt Psychology. New York, Harcourt, Brace. 1935.

12. Waisbren, B.A., Stern, M., and Collentine, G.E.: Methods of burn treatment. Comparison by probit analysis. JAMA 235: 255-58, 1975.

13. Hewitt, W.L. and Sanford, J.: Report of workshop held at NIH, Dec. 1972. J. Infec. Dis. 130:

14. Waisbren, B.A.: Meeting the challenge of critical care medicine. Wis. Med. J. 69: 197-200, 1970.

15. Waisbren, B.A., Simski, C., and Chang, P.: Administration of maximum doses of chloramphenicol. Am. J. Med. Sci. 245: 35-45, 1963.

16. Marquardt, M.: Paul Ehrlich. H. Schuman, Inc., 1951, p. 91

17. Waisbren, B.A.: Treatment with large doses of penicillin in a case of severe bacteremia due to Proteus. Arch. Int. Med. 91: 138-41, 1953.

18. Waisbren, B.A.: Intensive treatment of bone infections with antibiotics, intravenous gamma globulin, and aggressive therapy. Med. Counterpoint, Jan., 1970, pp. 23-32.

19. Waisbren, B.A. and Carr, C.: Penicillin and chloramphenicol in the treatment of infections due to Proteus organisms. Am. J. Med. Sci. 223: 418-21, 1952.

20. Jawetz, E.J., Gunnison, J.B., Speck, R.S., and Coleman, V.R.: Studies on antibiotic synergism and antagonism. Arch. Int. Med. 87: 349-59, 1951.

21. Lepper, M. and Dowling, H.F.: Treatment of pneumococcal meningitis with penicillin compared with penicillin plus aureomycin. Arch. Int. Med. 88: 489-94, 1951.

22. Waisbren, B.A.: The total management of the burned patient. J. St. Barnbas Med. Center 9: 1-10, 1972.

23. Waisbren, B.A.: Antibiotic treatment of bacterial endocarditis due to Enterococcus. Arch. Int. Med. 94: 846-52, 1954.

24. Simmons, H.E. and Strolley, P.D.: This is medical progress? Trends and consequences of antibiotic use in the United States. JAMA 227: 1623-28, 1974.

25. Scheckler, W.E. and Bennett, J.V.: Antibiotic usage in seven community hospitals. JAMA 213: 264-67, 1970.

26. Morgagni, Giovanni: De Salibus. 1761.

27. Pare, A.: The works of that famous chirurgian Ambrose Parey. Translated out of Latine and compared with the French by Thos. Johnson, London, Richard Cotes, and Willi Du-gard, 1649. Chapter 1, p. 1, as cited in Great Ideas in the History of Surgery - Zimmerman & Veith. Williams & Wilkins, 1961.

28. Waisbren, B.A.: An essay regarding pathogenesis and treatment of shock due to bacteremia with special reference to "gram-negative" shock. Progress in Cardiovascular Diseases, Vol. 10, No. 2, 1967. pp. 123-33.

29. Holden, W.D.: Professional agencies and the competence of physicians. JAMA 230: 441-42, 1974.

30. Federal Register. February 1975.

31. von Bertalanffy, L.: General System Theory. Foundations, Development, Applications. New York. George Braziller, Inc., 1969.

32. Waisbren, B.A.: Simultaneous multiple organ support. Paper presented at the Society for Critical Care Medicine, Anaheim, California, February 1974.

33. Waisbren, B.A.: Antibiotics in the treatment of burns. Surg. Clin. N. Amer. 50: 1311-23, 1970.

34. Waisbren, B.A., Martins, R.R., Bruns, W.T., and Kurzynski, T.A.: Whole cell heat-killed Gram-negative bacilli vaccine. Wis. Med. J. 73: 42-45, 1971.

35. Breitenbucher, R.B., et al.: Hepatorenal toxicity of tetracycline. Minn. Med. 53: 949-55, 1970.

36. Singhi, S., Waisbren, B.A., and Becker, I.M.: Granulomatous ileocolitis with multiple fistulae treated with gut rest, hyperalimentation, and anti-biotics. Wis. Med. J. 71: 152-54, May, 1972.

37. Tranquada, R.E., Bernstein, S., and Grant, W.J.: Intravenous methylene blue in the therapy of lactic acidosis. Arch. Int. Med. 114: 13-25, 1964.

38. Hermans, R.P.: Primary excision of full thickness burns up to 40% of body surface followed by micro- or meshgrafts. Research In Burns. Hans Huber, Vienna, 1971. Proc. 3rd Intl. Congress on Research in Burns. Prague, Sept., 1970, pp. 301-03.

39. Mueller, H., Evans, R., Religa, A. et al.: Nitroprusside effect on cardiac perfusion and metabolism in myocardial infarction. Circulation 50: No. 4: III-194, 1974.

40. Case Records of the Massachusetts General Hospital. N. Eng. J. Med. 284: 39-47, 1971.

41. Kreel, I., Osserman, K.E., Genkins, G., and Kark, A.E.: Role of thy-mectomy in the management of myasthenia gravis. Ann. Surg. 165: 111-17, 1967.

42. Schlegel, R.J.: Chronic granulomatous disease 1974. JAMA 231: 615-18, Feb., 1975.

43. Bortin, M.M., Saltzstein, E.C., Waisbren, B.A., Kay, S.A., Hong, R., Bach, R.H.: Bone marrow transplantation for aplastic anemia. Trans-plantation 12: 573-75, 1971.

44. Feng, P.H., et al.: Cyclophosphamide in treatment of systemic lupus ery-thematosus -- seven years' experience. Br. Med. J. 2: 450-52, 1973.

45. Chow, A.W., Forster, J., and Hryniuk, W.: Cytosine arabinoside therapy for Herpes virus infections. Antimicr. Agts. & Chemotherapy 70: 214-17, 1971.

46. Walker, W.W., Waisbren, B.A., Martins, R.R., and Batayias, G.R.: In vitro determinations of viral susceptibility to drugs for possible clinical use. Antimicro. Agts. & Chemotherap. 1970. pp. 380-84.

47. Waisbren, B.A.: The treatment of bacterial infections with the combination of antibiotics and gamma globulin. Antibiot. & Chemotherap. 7: 322-29, 1957.

242

48. McGowan, J.E., Jr., Garnier, C., Wilcox, C., and Finland, M.: Antibiotic susceptibility of Gram-negative bacilli isolated from blood cultures. Am. J. Med. 57: 225-38, 1974.

49. Helmholtz, H.V.: On thought in medicine. Address delivered in 1877 on the anniversary of the foundation of the Institute for Education of Army Surgeons. Reprinted from Bull of Instit. of History of Med. Johns Hopkins U. Press, 1938.

50. Arthus, Maurice: Philosophy of Scientific Investigation. Trans. by H.A. Sigerist. Baltimore. The Johns Hopkins U. Press. 1943.

51. Planck, Max K.E.L.: The Philosophy of Physics. New York, W.W. Norton, 1936.

52. Weiner, N.: Cybernetics. New York, John Wiley, 1948.

53. Shannon, C.: The mathematical theory of communication. Bell System Tech. J. 27: 80-84, April, 1950.

54. Snow, C.P.: The two cultures: and a second look. New York, Mentor, 1963.

55. Shoemaker, W.C., Elwyn, D.H., Levin, H., and Rosen, A.L.: Early prediction of death and survival in postoperative patients with circulatory shock by nonparametric analysis of cardiorespiratory variables. Crit. Care Med. 2: 317-25, 1974.

56. Shubin, H., Weil, M.H., Abdelmonem, A.A., Portigal, L., and Chang, P.: Selection of hemodynamic, respiratory and metabolic variables for evaluation of patients in shock. Crit. Care Med. 2: 326-36, 1974.

SIMULTANEOUS MULTIPLE ORGAN SUPPORT

Burton A. Waisbren, M.D., F.A.C.P.

Adapted from: Waisbren, B.A., Simultaneous Multiple Organ Support, Hospital Practice, May 1976, pp. 102-112.

244

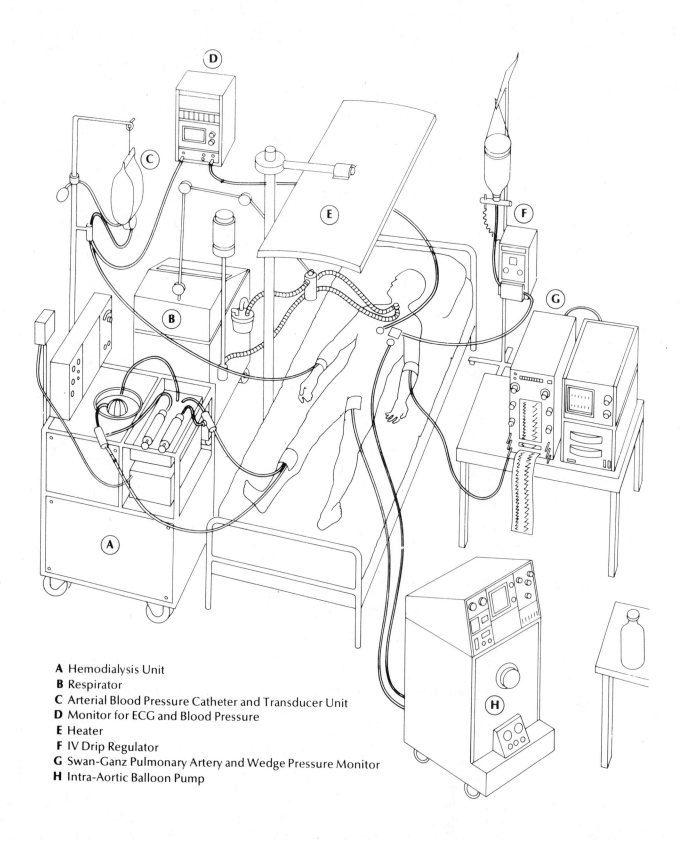

A Hemodialysis Unit
B Respirator
C Arterial Blood Pressure Catheter and Transducer Unit
D Monitor for ECG and Blood Pressure
E Heater
F IV Drip Regulator
G Swan-Ganz Pulmonary Artery and Wedge Pressure Monitor
H Intra-Aortic Balloon Pump

This figure is used with the kind permission of <u>Hospital Practice</u>, in which this article appeared, June 19, 1976.

Bedside observation in a critical care unit soon convinces one that patients seldom die of the failure of a single organ system. Multiple organ support, therefore, might very well result in the saving of a significant number of lives. This presentation is for those physicians whose experience has indicated a need for a system of multiple organ support and who are enthusiastic and energetic enough to try to develop such a system in their critical care units. This report delineates the components of the combined organ support system at the Burn Center and Critical Care Unit of St. Mary's Hospital in Milwaukee, Wisconsin, as a model for others. It also details exemplary case synopses and the specifics regarding the establishment of a combined organ support system.

ESSENTIAL COMPONENTS: Medicine is applied in so many different ways in the United States that the first emphasis in establishing a multiple organ support system must be on what is done--not on who does it. It matters not whether a nurse, medical resident, paramedic, or attending surgeon regulates the intra-arterial lines or the volume respirator, so long as it is done correctly and so long as the important decisions are made by the most highly trained members of the team, either on a contingency order basis or by direct communication[1,2]. In our unit the trained nurse, directed and backed up by the attending physicians, actually implements most changes in orders, but some units prefer physicians to be in attendance at all times during the acute phase of the illness. No matter who is chosen to be present, to advance to multiple organ support a unit must first incorporate into its daily routine the following: (1) the use of multiple arterial blood gas determinations; (2) direct measurement by transducers of arterial and venous pressures; (3) measurement of pulmonary artery and wedge pressures; (4) determination of cardiac output by thermodilution; (5) determination of levels and electrolytes, lactic acid, clotting elements, cortisol, blood volumes, weights, and colloid osmotic pressure[3]; (6) acute hemodialysis, with the ready availability of surgeons who can place good shunts; (7) a volume respirator in which PEEP is an easily added modality; (8) an intra-aortic balloon pump; and (9) a hyperbaric oxygen tank with a well trained crew[4,5]. As shown by our experience at St. Mary's Hospital, where these are all in operation, these modalities are all within the range of a moderate-size hospital. In fact, a good case can be made that every general hospital with an active emergency room must have all of these modalities for the adequate treatment of cases of myocardial infarction, poisonings, carbon monoxide poisoning, smoke inhalation, pulmonary failure, and severe trauma[5,6].

In addition to the machines mentioned above, the unit must have a widely used and understood drug tray, as outlined on Table 1, since each drug listed has possible indications that make its availability necessary for any attempt at multiple organ support[7-10].

SYNOPSES OF EXEMPLARY CASES

The following capsule descriptions are illustrative of the types of cases amenable to a multiple organ support system approach.

CASE 1: A 32-year-old male was burned over almost half of his body and suffered severe smoke inhalation. He was found unconscious in his burning bed and taken immediately to the hyperbaric chamber, where he was put under two atmospheres of oxygen for two hours. Carbon concentration in his blood at that time was 42 mg. %.

TABLE 1.   SOME OF THE DRUGS AND MEDICATIONS THAT SHOULD BE
AVAILABLE FOR MULTIPLE ORGAN SUPPORT

1. 20% ALBUMIN (7)*
2. AMINO ACIDS and GLUCOSE MIXTURE for HYPERALIMENTATION (27, 28)
3. AMPHOTERICIN B (27, 28)
4. CEDILANID (3)
5. CHLORAMPHENICOL (29)
6. DECADRON (30)
7. DEXTRAN (26)
8. DIBENZYLINE (PHENOXYBENZAMINE) (3, 15)
9. DILANTIN (22)
10. DOPAMINE (3-HYDROXYTRYAMINE) (19, 23)
11. GAMMA GLOBULIN (29)
12. GENTAMICIN (29, 36)
13. GLUCAGON (18)
14. ISUPREL (ISOPROTERENOL) (16)
15. LIDOCAINE (17)
16. METHICILLIN (29)
17. METHYLENE BLUE (33)
18. AMPULES OF NaHCarb (1, 3)
19. NOREPINEPHRINE (LEVOPHED) (3, 32)
20. PENICILLIN G (29)
21. FRESH FROZEN PLASMA (3)
22. PLATELET CONCENTRATE (3)
23. POLYMYXIN B (29)
24. PREMARIN (3)
25. PROPRANOLOL (INDEROL) (31)
26. TRIS (THAM) (3)

* References after each drug are for the reader who may be interested in
considering the modality for the drug tray in his Critical Care Department.

He then was transferred to the St. Mary's Burn Center, where he was found to be severely acidotic, in renal shutdown, with second and third degree burns over 42% of his body surface, and in shock (Table 2). The shock responded to an infusion of 250 mg. decadron and isuprel drip. After the first 24 hours his cardiovascular system remained intact. Admission ApO_2 was 40, so he was placed in a volume respirator (without PEEP) via an endotracheal tube. Volume respiratory assist was necessary for the next seven days. Eighteen hours after admission a shunt was placed in his right forearm. Hemodialysis was performed 19 times during the next 21 days, at which time his kidneys gradually started to regain normal function. During this time his burns were treated by the St. Mary's Burn Center System [11]. We removed his left arm because it was obviously mummified, and we gave him 17 units of cell mass for treatment of severe gastrointestinal hemorrhage. He made a steady recovery and when queried later said, "Yes, the treatment was worth it. I have never been fussed over so much in my life and I appreciate it."

COMMENT: This was the key case that showed us the feasibility of multiple organ support, hyperbaric oxygen, hemodialysis, and the volume respirator.

CASE 2: A 40-year-old woman was burned over 55% of her body and then lay at home, essentially unattended, for 48 hours. On admission she seemed remarkably intact, but within 24 hours it was apparent that she had suffered diffuse cell damage to her vital organs. Admission laboratory studies showed lactic acid of 5.6; blood urea nitrogen of 64; and nonsegmented polymorphonuclear cell percentage of 51 (viz., stab count) (Table 2). Arterial oxygen saturation, which was normal on admission, soon dropped to less than 32, and the entire lung developed patchy infiltration. Volume respiration was started through an endotracheal tube and a PEEP of 10, and this seemed to control the ApO_2 and general oxygenation. However, she became hypotensive, oliguric, and bacteremic in spite of decadron, heparinization, multiple antibiotics, 20% albumin, and isuprel. When her pulmonary wedge pressure had risen to 40/20 and her blood pressure could not be maintained above 50 mm. Hg. in spite of fluid, isuprel, cedilanid, and decadron, a single augmentation balloon was placed in her aorta. This was done without incident, and within one hour after balloon augmentation her blood pressure rose to 138/72 and she regained consciousness. Aortic counter pulsation was continued for 48 hours, after output had dropped markedly and her blood urea nitrogen was rising, so a shunt was placed and she was started on hemodialysis. Over the next 19 days she was dialyzed from two to four hours a day, maintained on hyperalimentation [9], treated with multiple antibiotics, and 33 cell mass transfusions were used to replace blood she lost--mostly by gastrointestinal bleeding. During all this time constant attempts were made to decrease the PEEP as a prelude to getting her off the respirator. These all were unsuccessful. She was fully conscious during this time and expressed the desire each day that we keep trying to do everything we could to help her. Her renal status and cardiovascular status seemed to stabilize, and her urine output started to come back. However, in spite of fresh frozen plasma, platelets, premarin, and small doses of heparin, she began to ooze from all sites and died in shock on the nineteenth day. In view of the bleeding and inability to wean her from the respirator, it was decided not to reinstitute aortic balloon augmention as her blood pressure fell for the final time.

TABLE 2.   SUMMARY OF THE IMPORTANT LABORATORY VALUES IN THE SIX REPORTED CASES

Time	Case 1	Case 2	Case 3	Case 4	Case 5	Case 6	Mean
			BUN VALUES				
Day 1	12	134	64	42	30	95	63 ± 41
Day 2	62	150	40	74	43	108	80 ± 39
Day 3	92	132	57	74	65	78	83 ± 24
Day 4	86	136	43	65	65	134	88 ± 35
			% STABS VALUES				
Day 1	33	56	29	21	34	25	33 ± 11
Day 2	56	41	26	55	19	32	38 ± 14
Day 3	2	2	27	40	49	8	21 ± 19
Day 4	21	4	23	--	62	72	30 ± 26
			PLATELET VALUES				Mean in Thous.
Day 1	530,000	101,000	112,000	176,000	240,000	15,000	196 ± 165
Day 2	101,000	70,000	81,000	130,000	98,000	16,000	83 ± 35
Day 3	52,000	54,000	64,000	50,000	42,000	42,000	47 ± 15
Day 4	87,000	43,000	10,000	----	26,000	7,500	35 ± 29
			FIBRINOGEN VALUES				
Day 1	270	730	620	170	185	175	358 ± 229
Day 2	570	600	830	98	210	---	462 ± 269
Day 3	380	145	590	72	170	310	278 ± 173
Day 4	345	205	680	---	---	455	421 ± 174
			ApO_2 VALUES				
Day 1	40.6	38.5	97.2	88.2	69.8	66.1	66.7 ± 22
Day 2	108.5	115.1	34.3	126.5	99.1	118.2	100.0 ± 31
Day 3	88.2	85.4	47.8	65.4	143.9	127.6	93.0 ± 33
Day 4	67.8	76.5	119.0	73.3	82.1	155.7	96.0 ± 32
			pH VALUES				
Day 1	7.17	7.35	7.44	7.13	7.20	7.47	7.29 ± 0.13
Day 2	7.54	7.49	7.54	7.40	7.10	7.42	7.41 ± 0.15
Day 3	7.56	7.47	7.55	7.35	7.37	7.40	7.45 ± 0.08
Day 4	7.51	7.47	7.54	---	7.37	7.43	7.46 ± 0.06
			LACTIC ACID				
Day 1	2.5	4.1	5.6	7.2	4.3	4.1	4.6 ± 1.5
Day 2	2.7	1.9	2.3	5.2	6.9	5.0	4.0 ± 1.8
Day 3	1.5	2.1	3.4	5.6	6.1	6.2	4.2 ± 1.9
Day 4	1.2	2.8	3.7	---	11.4	3.0	4.4 ± 3.6
			BLOOD VOLUME VALUES				
Day 1	54.1	95.0	87.9	64.1	59.2	85.9	76 ± 15
Day 2	60.8	65.3	83.5	49.9	49.7	89.6	66 ± 16
Day 3	60.1	61.7	103.6	48.0	55.0	81.0	68 ± 19
Day 4	59.3	76.6	90.8	---	78.6	81.0	77 ± 10

COMMENT: Autopsy showed most of her organs to be microscopically intact, with the exception of her lungs, which were essentially destroyed by infection, cellular necrosis, and cellular reaction.

CASE 3: A previously well 51-year-old woman was given an infusion of 5% dextrose in water that had become contaminated during manufacture. By the end of an elective procedure she was having hard shaking chills, hypotension, and tachycardia of 160. When seen two hours later she stated that she knew she was going to die. At that time her blood culture was positive for Escherichia coli, her ApO_2 was 50, her lactic acid was 8.4, her fibrinogen was 54, her blood pressure was 80/30, and her temperature was 106° F. Her cardiovascular system responded to maximum doses of cedilanid, isuprel, chloramphenicol, gentamicin, carbenicillin, and decadron, and within 12 hours she maintained a blood pressure of 80/70 and a very adequate urine output without any vasopressors[3]. However, within 48 hours she began to exhibit the classic x-ray picture of the "shocked lung," and when her ApO_2 dropped to 35 in spite of a volume respirator, she was transferred to St. Mary's Hospital for possible use of a membrane respirator. There an adequate ApO_2 was obtained with PEEP of 30, which she tolerated well in spite of subcutaneous emphysema. She became unconscious during this time but, aside from this, started to stabilize somewhat. She then went into complete renal shutdown, and daily hemodialysis was instituted to control her level of potassium, blood urea nitrogen, and blood volume. This was accomplished with daily eight-hour dialysis runs. The limiting factors seemed to be (1) an ability to wean her from the respirator; and (2) generalized bleeding due to disseminated vascular coagulation. She died in fairly good chemical balance on the sixteenth day of her illness.

COMMENT: The main feature of the autopsy was almost complete lack of functional lung tissue, with replacement by abscesses, exudate, and cellular debris. The family and staff felt, retrospectively, that the extreme efforts were justified, since each modality-volume respirator, transfer of the patient with an ApO_2 of 38, and hemodialysis--had been thoroughly weighed and discussed beforehand, and the patient was a strong, healthy woman prior to the tragic accident.

CASE 4: A 26-year-old male fell asleep smoking and was brought to the hospital deeply comatose, with second and third degree burns of over 95% of his body. Initial blood pH was 7.13, lactic acid was 7.2, and he was putting out very little urine (Table 2). Blood pressure was unobtainable. Initial resuscitation with 20 liters of Ringer's lactate and large amounts of NaHCarb, 250 mg. decadron, and 8 cc. cedilanid was successful, and 12 hours after admission he was semiconscious and had an arterial blood pressure of 80/60. Since he was in complete renal shutdown, a shunt was placed and hemodialysis was begun and used four hours daily for the remaining days of his life. He remained stable for about six hours, when his blood pressure began to fall in spite of norepinephrine, so he was taken to the operating room, where the aortic balloon was placed. He responded to the counter pulsation by regaining blood pressure, and during the next 24 hours he was stable. A tracheostomy was then done amid bleeding, because he had began to fight the endotracheal tube. The aortic balloon was then stopped, and 12 hours later he began to bleed in spite of fresh frozen plasma, heparin, premarin, platelets, and liberal transfusions. He then became hypotensive again. This time his blood pressure did not respond to the intra-aortic balloon pumping. At the time of death his lactic acid had fallen to 5.6 and all chemical tests were within acceptable limits (pH 7.35; ApO_2 66).

COMMENT: No apparent gross anatomical cause of death was apparent at autopsy. This patient was given vigorous treatment in spite of the almost total body burn because in the past we have saved patients with burns of this extent. All concerned, including the patient's family, were agreed that, at his age and with his previous excellent health, an all-out attempt should be made. The case certainly suggested to us the value of aortic balloon pumping in burn shock. When the patient's blood pressure is dropping steadily while he is on corticosteroids and norepinephrine, death is imminent; but his clinical condition was almost completely reversed after intra-aortic cardiac assist. Retrospectively we wonder if the augmentation should not have been continued for a longer period when it was first used and if tracheostomy might not have been performed earlier.

CASE 5: A 34-year-old male was brought in with third degree burns over 85% of his body suffered in a boiler explosion. He was alert and cooperative at the time of admission, and with 18 liters of fluid, decadron, endotracheal intubation, a volume respirator, cedilanid, and methylene blue he seemed to stabilize. However, 18 hours after admission he went into renal shutdown and his blood pressure fell to 40/0. After deliberation and discussion with him and his family, he was taken to the operating room where a double-barreled catheter for hemodialysis was placed in his vena cava and an aortic balloon was placed in his aorta. Hemodialysis and balloon pumping were begun immediately; his blood pressure rose to 160/100, his lactic acid fell somewhat, and his pH rose to 7.37. He maintained his improvement for the next 24 hours when, while on both dialysis and balloon augmentation, there was a rather sudden beginning of generalized bleeding. He became comatose and died from what looked like a central nervous system hemoorrhage.

COMMENT: Again, the response to the dialysis and balloon augmentation seemed to establish the potential value of this approach. The limiting factor apparently was the inability to control the generalized bleeding.

CASE 6: A 61-year-old man developed a Pseudomonas infection at the site of an angiogram, which had been done to rule out an aortic aneurysm. When seen first, three days after the operative procedure, his blood pressure was 40/0 (in spite of an isuprel drip), he was aneuric, his ApO_2 was 38, and he had a blue, mottled appearance. An endotracheal tube was placed and he was started on a volume respirator and given a fluid load--70 mg. dibenzyline, a levophed drip (10 mg. in 500 cc. D/5/W) to maintain his blood pressure at 70, 8 cc. cedilanid, 250 mg. decadron, 8 gm. chloramphenicol, 10 ml. gamma globulin, 80 mg. gentamicin, and 4 gm. carbenicillin. Rate of fluid administration was determined by the pulmonary artery wedge pressure. During the first 24 hours of the renal shutdown 3000 ml. of fluid were given. Within six hours the patient regained a systolic blood pressure. He was weaned from the norepinephrine within 12 hours. Only one dose of dibenzyline was given [3]. Eighteen hours after the renal shutdown a shunt was placed and hemodialysis was begun. This was done daily for seven days and then every other day for four days, at which time his kidneys regained enough function to return his essential blood urea concentration to normal. Time on the volume respirator was slightly more than 48 hours. All during this time he received 250 ml. 20% albumin every four hours. The most difficult part of the clinical management was severe bleeding from multiple stress ulcers, which were seen through a gastroscope. These were treated with 65 transfusions of cell mass, gastric thrombin, premarin, vitamin K, vasopressin, fresh frozen plasma, and platelet transfusions. The patient was totally unconscious for three days and definitely not very responsive for the next ten days, after which he became very alert. He stated firmly at that time, he "Never wanted anything like this to be done to me again. I remember every minute of the endotracheal tube and it was a horrible experience!" (We had thought he was unconscious.)

COMMENT: Four weeks later the patient ruptured a pancreatic cyst, suffered a myocardial infarction, and died, in full command of his mental faculties, while receiving the nonaggressive therapy he had requested.

GENERALIZATIONS FROM THE SIX SYNOPSES

Intractable bleeding (cases 2, 3, 4, and 5) and irreversible lung damage seemed to be the limiting factors in these cases. The most abnormal laboratory indicators were low platelet counts, low pH, and elevated lactic acid levels (Table 2). The bleeding could not be explained wholly on the basis of intravascular clotting. The two late deaths from lung destruction highlight the need for a better way of protecting this vital organ.

Lessons Derived from the Initial Cases of Multiple Organ Support

Based on the above patients and numerous others who have been on only one or two organ support systems, certain lessons have been learned. These include how best to organize a multiple organ support system in a general hospital and how to use each modality within the system.

ORGANIZATION: This depends on motivating the staff members of the entire hospital to use their often latent talents. We started out thinking that a "Renaissance man" type of effort, with one individual directing the volume respirator, artificial kidney, and aortic balloon pump as a kind of "Toscanini of the bedside", would be best. We soon learned that only by obtaining the participation of medical staff members with special interests and expertise in each element were we able to get a coordinated, enthusiastically functioning system. Thus an operating group consisting of the heads of the pulmonary department, hemodialysis, and cardiovascular surgery, the burn internist, and the burn surgeons, agreed upon criteria for the use of combined organ support. Now, when a physician in the hospital has a patient in need of multiple organ support, the ward communicator notifies the physicians on the rosters of the pulmonary, renal, cardiovascular surgery, and internal medicine departments, and each starts his elements of the system[2]. The head of each department reserves the right not to institute the modality in which he has the most experience. Since all these departments use the same critical care nurses as their paramedics, priorities and sequences seem to work out without undue difficulty. Each succeeding case seems to have run a little more smoothly, perhaps because in each case there has been general satisfaction at having taken part in a worthwhile endeavor. This satisfaction--and recognition of the role of each department--seems to us the element of the system that finally made it functional.

THE VOLUME RESPIRATOR: The limiting factor in getting a volume respirator assist for many patients who need it seems to be the lack of personnel who can insert an endotracheal tube. Enlisting the enthusiastic support of the anesthesiology department in backing up the critical care areas is a partial solution to this problem. However, it is possible that many more patients who need a volume respirator would be helped sooner if the respirator could be started automatically when certain criteria were met. To this end our anesthesiology department is now training our critical care nurses to put down endotracheal tubes. Once they are taught, they go to the operating room at least once a month to pass a tube under supervision, to keep up their proficiency. If they have difficulty, the anesthesiology department back-up is, of course, still available.

Tracheostomy should be done as early as possible, preferably while the patient is in the operating room, for the placing of the aortic balloon and the shunt. This is because bleeding and oozing will almost inevitably be a problem later in the course of illness, and having to do a tracheostomy when the patient is starting to recover in other ways often will tip the scales downward just when things are getting better (see Case 4). Early tracheostomy also makes aspiration of the pulmonary tree much easier and allows for accurate monitoring of the microorganisms that may be causing difficulties. Furthermore, it allows for easier use of the fiberoptic bronchoscope, which is rapidly becoming a sine qua non for keeping the lower respiratory tract clean of debris and exudate.

The use of PEEP on the volume respirator has increased the use and effectiveness of the respirator greatly. However, our experience would seem to indicate that PEEP should be used earlier than we have in the past, and that weaning should be as soon as possible. Also, PEEP seems to increase the spector of the adult respiratory syndrome. To prevent this we are exploring various methods of prophylaxis such as corticosteroids, albumin, and dilantin.

HEMODIALYSIS: The easy access to hemodialysis provided by a well-functioning multiple organ support system seems to have broadened the indications for its use considerably. In addition to its classical indications, hemodialysis appears to have a definite role in reducing the ever-present myocardial depressant factor in controlling blood pressure [12]. Furthermore, in the case of severe burns and immunodepressed patients, hemodialysis allows the use of full dosages of antiPseudomonas drugs such as polymyxin B and gentamicin, in spite of the fact they might temporarily shut down the kidneys (see Case 2) [9-11]. Hemodialysis has been of marked help in getting rid of sodium, particularly in the aged burn patient who often develops hypernatremia after being resuscitated with large amounts of Ringer's lactate [6]. Placing the shunt in the operating room at the same time the tracheostomy is being done and the balloon aortic pump is being inserted seems the most efficient way to be ready for exigencies such as fluid overload, hypernatremia, hyperkalemia, and antibiotic toxicities. Routine daily hemodialysis for the four or five days of extreme stress may prevent most of these conditions before they become clinically apparent.

INTRA-AORTIC AUGMENTATION OF CARDIAC OUTPUT, CARDIAC EMPTYING, AND CORONARY AND RENAL PERFUSION: Since the treatment of Case 6, balloon augmentation has changed from a relatively esoteric procedure to one of extensive use in cardiac intensive care units throughout the country. Apparently many others have shared our experience: that once the staff of a critical care unit becomes familiar with the procedure it is relatively simple, obviously lifesaving in many instances, and does not require the constant presence of a physician[13]. Implementation of balloon pumping in a unit is best made as an extension of an open heart surgery program. The biomedical engineer involved in maintaining the bypass for open heart surgery can train the nurses or pump technicians in the monitoring of balloon pumping in a three- to four-hour course, and then the critical care nurse can monitor the pump as long as she has good telephone back-up with the physicians or even with the open heart surgery pump technicians.

The balloon is best inserted at the same time the hemodialysis shunt, tracheostomy, and flow-directed catheters are being placed (see above). Experience in our unit and elsewhere seems to indicate an ever-lengthening time during which the pump can be used, but at present our protocol calls for a standard 48-hour run. If, thereafter, the cardiac output is still unsatisfactory and survival still seems possible, a much longer time is indicated and can be tolerated by many patients[13]. In our most recent cases we have found it necessary to turn off the pump on several occasions, while the patient either received hyperbaric oxygen treatment or had ruptured stomach ulcers repaired. During these intervals the clotting time was kept at between 20 and 30 minutes (Lee-White) by heparin, and no untoward results seemed to occur. Whereas with PEEP our concept is becoming "start earlier and stop earlier", with the balloon aortic pump our current thinking is "start sooner and continue longer." Based on the current literature regarding cardiac shock, it seems this modality will soon be used much more commonly than it has been in the past[13]. Cardiac surgeons have been the logical individuals to set up and institute balloon pumping in a critical care unit, and success may well be a function of the close involvement of these surgeons in this endeavor. On the other hand, the apparatus is simple enough so that an interested vascular surgeon who may not be involved in open heart work should have no trouble in setting up the procedure.

HYPERBARIC OXYGEN: The proven efficacy of hyperbaric oxygen in the treatment of gas gangrene, carbon monoxide poisoning, and industrial "bends", and the probable effectiveness of this modality in burn care and treatment of recalcitrant cases of osteomyelitis; and its possible use in many other conditions make the availability of hyperbaric oxygen a necessity in every large community. The smaller hyperbaric chambers are relatively simple and inexpensive. When new cases of smoke inhalation were treated in a walk-in chamber 20 miles from St. Mary's Burn Center, we found the logistics unacceptable from the standpoint of applying our usual critical care system. Therefore, a chamber was purchased and made operative under the direction of the pulmonary service of the hospital. An experienced critical care nurse and five licensed pulmonary therapists were trained by the director of this department, and a call system was devised through which patients could be given hyperbaric oxygen with a minimum of confusion and delays*. The more routine use of hyperbaric oxygen in burn cases[14] and in cases of difficult osteomyelitis provided the in-service training needed for keeping up the staff's hyperbaric oxygen proficiency.

* The Procedure Manual for the tank hyperbaric chamber, written by Dr. Edward Banaszak, is available on request to him at St. Mary's Hospital.

DISCUSSION

What is the indication for multiple organ support? Simply stated, it can be described as any situation in which a patient will probably die of multiple organ failure and in which his physician feels justified in going "all out" to save him. Since all of the modalities used are accepted forms of treatment, their use in combination should not be considered extraordinary or investigative treatment and should require no special permission or committee regulation.

Multiple organ support is indicated in four main types of patients: (1) the young individual with burns over 80% of his body; (2) patients in gram-negative shock; (3) patients in cardiogenic shock who are either being prepared for surgery or who are potentially salvageable but are not surgical candidates; and (4) young patients with the adult respiratory syndrome. How the physician makes his decision to undertake the effort must be influenced by prior discussion with colleagues, with the patient himself, if possible, and with his family. Once the decision is made, however, the team must be made operative and start to function without delay. We use a single ward communicator who notifies the person in charge of each department, who, in turn, notifies the person on call for his department.

Once the machines are placed and running it is surprising how simple it is to keep them coordinated. This is done by daily manipulations by the representatives of each service. One physician writes daily fluid and medication orders and goals for kidney, lung, and heart function. Remarks such as, "Let's take off some fluid and replace it with red blood cells during the dialysis" or "The sooner we get off the PEEP the quicker we can reduce out balloon pumping," made either in person or on the chart, give guidance to the chest and renal service representatives. We find this kind of interplay works better at the higher levels of each service than among individuals in residency training.

Knowing that multiple organ support can be accomplished successfully in the general hospital setting should stimulate many physicians, who are responsible for the types of patients we have described, to develop a system. Although the more carefully planned the system is, the better it will eventually become, the best way to initiate development of a system of multiple organ support is probably for a group of dedicated physicians to evolve it while working on a particular patient whom they are determined to save. Each success or failure in this framework seems to add elements to a system which are beneficial the next time it becomes necessary to use it. Furthermore, under the extreme tension of caring for the mortally ill patient, solutions and compromises between the different disciplines involved seem easier to reach than they are within a distant conference room.

There are fringe benefits to developing a multiple organ support in a hospital that might compensate for the fact that it requires a very high investment in time and equipment for relatively rare use. First, each separate modality is essential for any hospital that wishes to operate a modern emergency service. Second, the degree of finesse and the exchange of information necessary to develop a multiple organ support system cannot fail to increase the effectiveness of each separate component. From the standpoint of staff morale and pride, the endeavor is also worthwhile. It is a great feeling for all who are involved to realize they can function as a team to salvage a patient who is otherwise fated to die from the emergency condition that brought him to the hospital.

REFERENCES

1. Waisbren, B.A.: <u>Critical Care Manual: A Systems Approach Method.</u> Medical Examination Publishing Co., Inc., Flushing, N.Y., 1972.

2. Waisbren, B.A.: Care of the critically ill: the systems method. The Hospital Medical Staff 1: Feb., 1972.

3. Waisbren, B.A.: Meeting the challenge of critical care medicine. Wis. Med. J. 69: 197-200, 1970.

4. Editorial: Intra-aortic balloon counterpulsation: a weaning assist. JAMA 224: 1183, 1973.

5. Meijne, N.G., Mellink, H.M., and Kox, C.: The main present-day indications for clinical treatment in a hyperbaric chamber. Pneumonoligic 149: 173-180, 1973.

6. Chamion, H., et al.: Indications for early hemodialysis in multiple trauma. Lancet 1: 1125-1127, 1974.

7. Holzer, J., Karliner, J.S., O'Rourke, R.A., et al.: Effectiveness of dopamine in patients with cardiogenic shock. Am. J. Cardiol. 32: 79-84, 1973.

8. Waisbren, B.A.: Intensive treatment of bone infections with antibiotics, intravenous gamma globulin, and aggressive therapy. Med. Counterpoint 2: 23-32, 1970.

9. Singhi, A., Waisbren, B.A., and Becker, I.M.: Granulomatous ileocolitis with multiple fistulae treated with gut rest, hyperalimentation, and antibiotics. Wis. Med. J. 71: 152-154, 1972.

10. Law, D.K., Dudrick, S.J., and Abdous, N.I.: Immunocompetence of patients with protein calorie malnutrition. Ann. Int. Med. 74: 545-549, 1972.

11. Waisbren, B.A.: The total management of the burned patient. J. St. Barnabas Med. Center 9: 1-10, 1972.

12. Vaisrub, S.: Myocardial depressant factor (MDF) in cardiogenic shock. JAMA 228: 500, 1974.

13. Mathivat, A., Bourdarias, J.P., Bardet, J., et al.: Prolonged circulatory assistance by intra-aortic unidirectional counter pulsation in a state of shock following myocardial infarction. La Nouvelle Presse Medical 2: 2663-2667, 1973.

14. Hart, G.B., Thompson, R.E., Depenbush, F.L.: The treatment of thermal burns with hyperbaric oxygen: A retrospective study. J. St. Barnabas Med. Center 9: 16-19, July, 1972.

DRUG INDEX